A WOMAN'S ADDICTION WORKBOOK

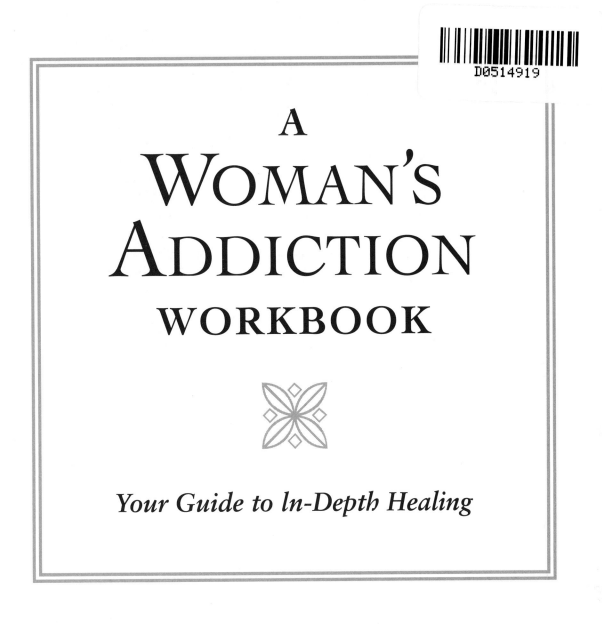

Your Guide to In-Depth Healing

LISA M. NAJAVITS, PH.D.

NEW HARBINGER PUBLICATIONS, INC.

Publisher's Note

This publication is designed to provide accurate and authoritative information in regard to the subject matter covered. It is sold with the understanding that the publisher is not engaged in rendering psychological, financial, legal, or other professional services. If expert assistance or counseling is needed, the services of a competent professional should be sought.

Distributed in Canada by Raincoast Books

Copyright © 2002 by Lisa M. Najavits
New Harbinger Publications, Inc.
5674 Shattuck Avenue
Oakland, CA 94609

Cover design by Poulson/Gluck Designs

ISBN-10 1-57224-297-3
ISBN-13 978-1-57224-297-5

Printed in the United States of America

New Harbinger Publications' website address: www.newharbinger.com

09   08   07

15   14   13   12   11   10   9   8   7   6

To my grandmother, Margot E. Kolan, who told me, "Be the leader, not follower, of your life." And for all that she overcame.

Contents

Part II
Healing

Acknowledgments

Thanks to the following people:

For their dedication to improving women's treatment and their support of my work: Vivian Brown, Sharon Cadiz, Pamela Detrick, Norma Finkelstein, Jean Harvey, Denise Hien, Holly Hills, Frances Hutchins, Beth Glover Reed, Robert Rosenheck, Joseph Ruzek, Beth Weinman, and Caron Zlotnick.

For mentorship on my research studies: Roger Weiss and Howard Shaffer.

For their wonderful writing on women's addiction and their generosity: Stephanie Covington, Charlotte Kasl, Betsy McCaul, and Joan Zweben.

Margaret Cramer and Arthur Klein, for some fascinating conversations.

My writers' group: Deirdre Barrett, Judah Lebland, Ian Ruderman, Jess Steigerwald, Deborah Strod, and Andrew Szanton.

My husband, Burke Nersesian, for the immense joy of being able to come home to him at the end of the day.

My clients, whose struggles have moved me.

Catharine Sutker of New Harbinger Publications, for suggesting this book.

Finally, to the promise of the future. While treatment has improved in the past twenty years, there are still far too many women with addiction who feel alone and unhelped.

PART I

Exploration

INTRODUCTION

Starting Out

This book is designed to help you overcome an addiction. The focus will be substance addiction, which is the most well known addiction in women. However, you may find the strategies relevant to other addictions as well, including food, television, work, Internet, relationships, gambling, sex, exercise, or any other area of your life that is out of control.

This book is designed to be your companion—to help you explore your addiction and to encourage your best self to emerge. At this point, you may not even be sure you have a real problem. Perhaps you are just wondering about addiction, or others may have told you they think you have a problem. That's fine—part of the exploration will be to figure it out for yourself. If you find you do have a problem, you can then explore how you want to go about working on it.

The book was written to be relevant to as many women as possible. It does not assume a particular type of woman, nor a particular substance. It seeks to draw together material in an inclusive way that, hopefully, will inspire you to improve your life. You do not have to feel that you are highly feminine, a feminist, or that you identify strongly with women. (Indeed, some women feel more allied with men.) You may have a mild, moderate, or severe addiction. You may be in treatment or not.

You may wonder how a book can apply to so many different women. The reason is simple: While each woman has her own unique history, recovery can be boiled down to one common task. The task is simple but not easy: *to learn to respect who you are*. It's impossible to both truly respect yourself and continue an addiction you know is destroying you. Respect at the deepest level means valuing yourself—it may involve taking care of your body, finding healthy relationships, reducing stress, getting treatment, facing the pain of the past, or making use of supports in your community. It is often a mix of these strategies and many more. You likely have heard of such solutions, but getting yourself to do them may have felt impossible. This book seeks to help you summon the energy and courage for the work.

Throughout, you will be guided to take steps to help yourself, and it will be up to you to choose what they are. Methods that work for one woman may not work for another. You may want to read about addiction, work on the skills in this book, seek therapy, attend 12-step groups such as Alcoholics Anonymous (AA), or go into the hospital, for example. This book does not advocate one solution over any other, but views all as possibilities. There are as many roads to recovery as there are to addiction. Each woman has her own path.

There is a natural tendency to feel like a failure if you have an addiction. You may hear this from others as well: "Don't you see what you've done to the family?" or "You would stop if you really wanted to." But it's known that addictions go much deeper—it's not simply a matter of willpower or "pulling yourself up by your boot-straps." Self-blame and guilt don't solve the problem. What solves it is gentle understanding and supportive action.

A key message in this book is that there are understandable reasons why you became addicted. These may include life issues that felt overwhelming, such as relationship conflicts, a history of violence or trauma, emotional problems, poverty, or a work life that is too stressful. They may include biological vulnerability, such as a family history of addiction; or societal forces, such as frequent contact with people who use substances. Whatever the reason—and typically it is not one, but many—you can explore how to heal now, how to stop the downward spiral that addiction inevitably becomes.

There is a self deep inside who is wise, kind, and strong—your best self. Addiction may have obscured that deepest self, or you may find that your best self is only present at certain moments. But the goal now is to get back to her. You may have come to view your addiction as who you are, but it's not. Someday you'll be able to look back at your addiction as a small part of your identity. You can have a full, rich life. You may not believe this right now—that's okay. It's part of addiction to doubt that the future can be different.

Identify, if you can, a "best self" you're going to try to create, to take back from the addiction. Perhaps it's an image of who you want to become—someone who runs her own business or raises her kids sober. Perhaps it's an image of who you were at a younger age, before the addiction took hold—more innocent or joyful. Identify that best self and keep her in mind as you go through this book. The issues that have obscured her can be overcome. Your real self, your right to a life that is genuine and meaningful, still exists no matter how many years you've been addicted.

Feel free to skip around to whatever interests you; there's no order to be followed. You can do the second half of the book (Healing) before the first half (Exploration). If you benefit from reading a page every day, do that. If you prefer just browsing as you feel inspired, do that. Let your process with this book mirror the process of healing: to respect your intuition about where you need to go. You have a natural ability to heal if given enough guidance and freedom to look at yourself without judgment. The key is to understand yourself at a deeper level. Behind all addiction there is a good person who got off track. You can find your way back. Many have, and you can too.

You can also use this book in connection with any current treatment you attend, such as therapy or self-help groups. You can let people know what areas you are working on, and seek their feedback.

It's suggested that you repeat the exercises in part II of this book as often as you can. Practice using real-life situations. With time and persistence, it can become natural to live differently.

If you become very upset while reading any part of this book, find a professional therapist or counselor in your community. Some of the topics may stir feelings that have been pushed away for a long time. While the goal is not to make you upset, it could happen. The priority is safety. If you get very depressed, feel you want to die or hurt yourself, or become aggressive toward others, seek help. Remember you never have to be alone with what you are going through.

If you have been using a substance frequently or in large amounts (such as several drinks per day), it's strongly recommended that you obtain a doctor's assistance in coming off the substance. For some substances, such as pills or heroin, you may need medical monitoring.

Throughout the book, the term "women" will be used, but the material can be applied to girls under eighteen years of age as well. Unless otherwise noted, the information is based on substance abuse; however, it may also be relevant to other addictions. There are many terms for addiction: substance abuse, dependence, alcoholism, chemical dependency, substance use disorder. In this book, *addiction* is used in as broad a sense as possible. In chapter 2, definitions will be discussed.

Finally, note that this book was developed to help women explore issues specific to them. If you are new to recovery, you may also want to read more generally on addiction. Resources are provided in many of the chapters.

Most of all, the message is: there is hope. Often by the time the addiction has taken hold, so too has hopelessness about your life. You may feel your life is already ruined, that you might as well keep using, that you're in too deep to get out, that you don't have what it takes. If you remember one idea from all the pages in this book, let it be this: you can recover. Keep reading and stay open to what you might find. For now, just turn the page. . . .

CHAPTER 1

Why a Book for Women?

You may be wondering why there is a need for a woman's addiction book. Don't the principles of recovery apply equally to men and women? Also, women are not all alike, so perhaps it's not possible to focus on them as a group.

When I began in the addiction field, I wondered about these issues too. However, in ten years of treating women and conducting research, I have come to understand—to truly "get"—that there are indeed key differences between women and men in addiction. How and why addictions begin, their course, and their recovery may all vary based on gender.

Until recently, the vast majority of addiction work was based on men. It was assumed that whatever held true for men would apply as well to women (Brady and Randall 1999). The 12-step movement was founded by men; treatment programs were designed for men; assessment and research focused on men; and until the past decade or two, women's programs did not exist. Indeed, this bias toward men occurred throughout health care, not just in the addiction field (Blumenthal 1998).

Recently, however, it has been recognized that women differ from men in their health care needs. As Goldberg (2002) says, "Women are not small men." You will see in this chapter that women with addiction differ dramatically from men in many ways. Thus, the good news is that there is now greater awareness of women's issues and a wider variety of treatment options than ever before. Recent progress includes the adaptation of 12-step and other recovery resources for women, and the development of new treatments such as women-and-children programs and gender-based services (Covington 2000; Kasl 1992; McCaul and Svikis 1999). Much work remains to be done, but the idea that women are like men is no longer just assumed. Indeed, all federally funded studies now require that females be included.

Why was addiction treatment initially focused on men? There are several reasons. First, men have much higher rates of addiction than women, a pattern consistent across societies and across time (Fillmore et al. 1997). Thus, it makes sense that the addiction field focused first on this most prominent group. Second, men's problems were often more visible. Until a few decades ago, women's role was in the home while men's was in the public workplace. Women's addiction could be largely ignored. Due to greater social stigma for women—the view that it was fine for men to drink but not for women—there was even more reason for women's addiction to be hidden (Gomberg and Nirenberg 1993). Women also sought addiction treatment less (Greenfield, in press- b). Third, and not least, men have held more power in society. It used to be said that it was a "man's world," and thus women's issues, in addiction as elsewhere, took a backseat. Only with the recent women's rights movement has this bias begun to be corrected.

Would you like to understand more about gender issues in addiction? If so, read the next section, which describes "the good news and the bad news." Later in this chapter, you can read about rates of addiction in women, the different types of women with addiction, and the personal story of one woman who achieved thirty years clean and sober from substances. You will be guided, if you want, to tell your own story as well. A list of free resources on addiction appears at the end of the chapter.

The Good News and the Bad News

The good news is that women have lower rates of addiction than men, and they are more likely than men to benefit from treatment. The bad news is that women are much more likely to suffer serious negative effects from addiction, even if they use less and start at a later age. They are also less likely to get support for their recovery and more likely to have emotional difficulties in addition to addiction. Women's rate of addiction is increasing at a fast pace, especially among young women and girls.

The summary in this section is based on a wide review of research. If you want a quick summary, skim the section headings; if you like details, read the whole thing. If you're someone who "tunes out" factual information, just read whatever interests you. Note that this is the chapter with the most facts. Starting in the next chapter, we'll explore more about *you*—your history, current situation, feelings, and thoughts.

The Good News

When women seek help for their addiction, they can succeed in forging a new and better life. This is good news indeed. Some specifics follow.

Women respond better to treatment than men. Women's substance use decreased twice as much as men's in a recent national study of thousands of addicts five years after treatment (SAMHSA 1998). Moreover, they are more likely to remain abstinent once they enter treatment (Weiss et al. 1997), are more likely to complete substance abuse treatment (Wallen 1998), and are more likely to respond to outpatient behavioral treatment (McCrady and Raytek 1993). Even in adolescence, girls are more likely to respond to addiction treatment than boys (McCrady and Raytek 1993). When given treatment, women show major decreases in drug use and criminal arrests (SAMHSA 1997). Finally, if women attempt moderate drinking, they are more likely to be successful than men (McCrady and Langenbucher 1996).

New programs sensitive to women are being developed. Knowledge is growing about how best to treat women with addiction. Programs are starting to address the multiple needs of women—including trauma histories, co-occurring disorders such as depression and anxiety, parent training, job training, medical care, and domestic violence—rather than just providing treatment for the addiction itself (Finkelstein 1993). A notable advance has been the development of women-focused addiction treatment, which, at least in initial studies, has been found to improve success rates compared to mixed-gender treatment (Blume 1998). In general, while addiction treatment was not very effective for many years, in the past decade improved treatments of all kinds have led to higher success rates (Miller et al. 1995; Najavits and Weiss 1994).

Treating women effectively can have a positive impact on their children. Addiction programs designed to address the needs of pregnant women have had a positive impact on both the new mothers and their children (Clark 2001). If a substance-abusing woman receives treatment, the cost of health services for her child in the first two years of life are 1.4 times lower than if she does not receive treatment; this is not only an economic saving, but a direct way to prevent health care problems in children. If a woman is able to keep custody of her children, she is also more likely to succeed in treatment (Drug Strategies 1998). Similarly, if women are allowed to keep their children with them during residential treatment, they are less likely to drop out and are more successful after treatment (Coletti et al. 1997).

Women have more awareness of substance abuse issues than men. More women view addiction as a serious problem in their communities and among young people. Women are more likely to view treatment as a positive step for people who have problems. Women are more supportive of funding addiction programs, of needle-exchange programs, and of testing drivers for substances. Women are also more likely to talk to their children about substances and to believe their children can obtain them (Drug Strategies 1998; Greenfield, in press-a).

The Bad News

Unfortunately, the list of bad news is longer. You're taking an important step by reading this—hopefully, it will energize you to take on your recovery with enthusiasm and commitment. Sometimes a "wake-up call" is what's needed to start off on a new path. Knowing the realities of women and addiction may help you see more clearly what you need to do for yourself.

If, however, you become very upset while reading this section, you can skip it. In later chapters, we'll discuss how to take *any* negative feeling and help make it work for you. But for now, just seek to protect yourself if you need to. Some women early in recovery prefer to focus on positives; they don't want to hear bad news. That's fine too—it means you're taking care of yourself.

Women are more likely to die from addiction than men. Women are twice as likely to die from alcohol-related problems as men (McCrady and Raytek 1993). Women who abuse substances are more likely to attempt suicide than men (Blume 1997b). Women are three times more likely to die from lung cancer as men who smoke the same amount (Brody1998). AIDS (typically from injection drug use) is one of the leading causes of death among young women (Selwyn 1998). Did you know that the number of women dying from illnesses related to addiction is *more than four times* the number who die from breast cancer (Blumenthal 1998)? Yet there is far less attention to addictions in the media and society. When was the last time you saw a fund-raising walk for women's addiction treatment? Addiction truly is a life-or-death issue for women. It's been called a "silent epidemic" because it's been hidden and neglected for so long (Drug Strategies 1998).

Women become addicted more quickly than men. For example, even though women generally drink less than men, they progress more quickly into alcoholism. This means that it takes fewer years for females to go from their first experience of intoxication, to problem drinking, to treatment. This is called a *telescoped course*, which means rapid progression from using to abusing (Piazza, Vrbka, and Yeager 1989).

Women are more likely to develop health problems from addictions than men. The list is frightening: women alcoholics are more likely to suffer liver disease, cognitive impairment, and physical injury. They also more quickly develop anemia, malnutrition, hypertension, and peptic ulcer from alcohol. Alcoholism is known to lead to breast cancer, pancreatitis, cardiovascular problems, and gynecologic problems (Blume 1997b; NIAAA 2001). In fact, *just two drinks a day* puts women at high risk for physical illness, while for men it's five drinks a day (Greenfield 2002). Why the difference? Women's bodies process alcohol differently. (This is due to the influence of female hormones, different processing of alcohol in the stomach, less water in women's bodies, and more body fat.) After drinking the same amount, women have more alcohol in their blood. Because the alcohol is more concentrated, it does more damage to body organs (Gomberg and Nirenberg 1993).

Women are less likely to seek addiction treatment than men. Many women may not feel comfortable in treatment, which historically was designed for men. Women sometimes fear that if their addiction problem is known, their children will be taken away or they will be judged harshly. They also may not know they have an addiction problem, as they are less likely to be diagnosed than men (Blume 1997b). When they do seek help, they go to their medical doctors or to the mental health system more than to substance abuse treatment programs; but these avenues may not provide adequate attention to addiction (Moras 1998). Indeed, Blume concludes that the treatment needs of women with addictions "are still largely unmet" (1997b, 645).

Women are imprisoned at higher rates than ever before, primarily due to substances. This includes arrests for drug possession; crimes committed to support addiction, such as theft or prostitution; and sale of drugs. The past decade saw one of the largest increases ever in women serving sentences, largely due to mandatory sentencing laws in response to the crack cocaine epidemic in the 1980s. Women in the criminal justice system tend to have histories of physical and/or sexual abuse, often served as low-level associates to men who trafficked in drug sales, and are typically nonviolent offenders (Battle et al., in press).

Women have more barriers to treatment than men. Women are known to have a harder time entering addiction treatment due to child-care pressures, lack of money, and transportation problems (Schober and Annis 1996). They're also less likely to be encouraged to go to treatment by family and friends (Beckman and Amaro 1986). Pregnant substance-abusing women may be jailed or lose custody of their children. In medical settings, women are less likely to be identified as having addiction than men (Chang 1997), and assessment procedures appear less accurate for women than for men (Mendelson and Mello 1998). Some women fear separation from their children and lack of day care if they enter treatment (Coletti 1998).

Women are judged more harshly for addiction than men. This has been true throughout history and remains so today. A woman may be labeled a "lush," a "bad mother," or sexually "loose," while a man is viewed as "just one of the guys" (Heath 1993). A man sitting at a bar is seen differently than a woman. One survey shows that even women alcoholics view women's intoxication as "more obnoxious and disgusting" than men's (Gomberg and Nirenberg 1993). This double standard has existed for a long time in Western culture. Women were expected to drink less and not become drunk in public. Indeed, they were expected to uphold moral virtue and control men's drunkenness, while their own addiction was typically ignored (Nadeau and Harvey 1995). Such social stigma may make it harder for women to seek help.

Women tend to take on the addiction patterns of their partners, while men do not. For example, a woman involved with someone who drinks heavily is likely to start drinking more. Moreover, women entering addiction treatment are more likely to have a male partner with an addiction problem, while men entering treatment are more likely to have a nonaddicted partner (Blume 1997b).

Women with addiction become more socially isolated than men. They drink at home alone more and are more socially rejected. One study showed that 84 percent of alcoholic women did their drinking at home (Blume 1997b). Also, they have more family problems related to addiction (Gomberg and Nirenberg 1993).

Women with addiction have more emotional problems than men. These include depression, anxiety, eating disorders, and posttraumatic stress disorder, for example. Women also have lower self-esteem (McCrady and Raytek 1993). These are clear findings shown over and over again in research. Women suffer more emotional problems, while men experience more problems in functioning (e.g., work, money, and legal problems) (Gomberg and Nirenberg 1993). Unfortunately, women tend to receive inadequate treatment for emotional problems. They may just be referred to Alcoholics Anonymous rather than also being evaluated for psychiatric medication or therapy; this can lead to a much longer addiction problem. Notably, the emotional problem usually occurs first, and the addiction second—suggesting "self-medication," in which the woman tries to cope by using a substance (Kandel 1998).

Women's addiction is associated with reproductive problems. This includes increased risk of spontaneous abortion, early menopause, difficulty becoming pregnant, and changes to the period and ovulation (Blume 1997b). If a woman drinks while pregnant, she may give birth to a child with fetal alcohol syndrome, a set of abnormalities that can hinder the child for life. Substance abuse is the most widespread problem in high-risk pregnancies (Woods 1998). Many pregnant women avoid contact with the medical community because they are afraid their children will be taken away; thus, prenatal care is missed.

Women's substance use is increasing. Young women are using substances at higher rates than ever before (Blumenthal 1998). Teen girls' drinking and smoking are increasing more than that of teen boys. Women's use of cocaine, opiates, and nicotine rose in the 1990s, while men's did not. Women's use of multiple substances (polysubstance use) is also on the increase. In the past decade, the number of emergency room visits related to heroin and marijuana rose more for women than for men (Drug Strategies 1998; Miller 1999).

Girls are trying substances at increasingly younger ages. In the past three decades, teen girls have been experimenting with substances at increasingly younger ages.

Indeed, by the early 1990s, girls' age of first alcohol use was for the first time the same as boys' (Greenfield, in press- b). Unfortunately, the younger a child experiments with substances, the more likely she is to become dependent later in life. "Every year that drug use is prevented buys important time for personal growth and intellectual development" (Drug Strategies 1998, 8). For example, if teens begin drinking before age fifteen, they are four times more likely to develop alcoholism than if they begin at age twenty-one. The same is true for smoking. One in three girls who tries cigarettes becomes a regular smoker; if they get to age twenty-one without smoking, however, it is unlikely they'll ever become addicted (Drug Strategies 1998).

Women are the fastest growing group of new HIV cases, largely due to drugs. During the past decade, new HIV cases decreased among men but increased among women. Among teens, girls' rate of HIV infection is increasing more than boys. Sixty-five percent of women who get HIV contract it from injection drug use or sexual contact with someone who injects drugs (Blumenthal 1998). AIDS is now the third leading cause of death in women of reproductive age, and the first among African-American women in that age group. Women with HIV who use drugs are also at increased risk for sexually transmitted diseases, gynecologic infections, and cervical abnormalities compared to those who don't use drugs (Selwyn 1998).

Women receive less emotional support from their partners for entering treatment. When women enter treatment, their partners tend to remain neutral; when men enter treatment, their partners tend to be highly supportive. Also, women are more often left by a partner for drinking than men. A common saying is that "90 percent of alcoholic women and 10 percent of alcoholic men are divorced" (Gomberg and Nirenberg 1993, 133). While overstated, it speaks to this point.

Many addicted women suffered violence, yet most never receive treatment for it. Among women in substance abuse treatment, 55 to 99 percent experienced trauma, typically childhood physical or sexual abuse, domestic violence, or rape. Thirty-three to 59 percent currently have posttraumatic stress disorder (PTSD) resulting from such experiences, which can endure for decades unless it's treated. For men in substance abuse treatment, rates of PTSD are two to three times lower (Najavits, Weiss, and Shaw 1997). Yet treatment for trauma remains rare: most substance abuse programs do not assess, treat, or educate patients about trauma (Najavits, 2002). It's also known that the more violence a woman endures, the more serious her addiction problem. Trauma victims have high rates of depression, self-mutilation, and suicidal impulses, and other, nonsubstance addictions are common, including eating disorders, abusive relationships in adulthood, sexual addiction, and compulsive exercise (Kilpatrick, et al. 1998). Sadly, addiction predisposes women to more trauma in the future (e.g., going home with a stranger after drinking). The link between trauma and use of hard drugs—cocaine and opiates—is also well known (Najavits, Weiss, and Shaw 1997).

Women are just as likely as men to have genetic vulnerability to substance abuse. Research shows that a tendency to become addicted may be inherited. Indeed, if you have a family history of addiction, you're 2.5 times more likely to develop it than someone without this background (Merikangas 1998). Family history is one of the single most important influences on who develops addiction. This is just as true for women as for men. However, it's important to emphasize that genetic vulnerability does not mean you can't recover: if you work at recovery, you too can succeed.

Women's substance use is associated with sexual problems. Sexuality and substance use have been linked throughout history (Kandall 1998). Many women report more interest and enjoyment in sex after using. Heavy use, however, can lead to sexual problems. When using substances, people are also more likely to engage in risky sexual practices that lead to disease and unwanted pregnancy. Some women are only able to engage in sex when using a substance, and thus become addicted as this pattern gets entrenched over time (Gomberg and Nirenberg 1993).

Some addictions are more common in women than men. Women are more likely to abuse tranquilizers and sleeping pills (Graham and Braun 1999). They're more likely to become regular users of cocaine after a shorter period of time, and they report shorter abstinent periods (White, Brady, and Sonne 1996). Women are more likely to have dependence on physical exercise (Pierce, Rohaly, and Fritchley 1997), although this has only recently been studied. At every age, women are more likely to get addicted to tobacco, and smoking is more likely to lead to drug abuse for women than for men. Smoking among women is often associated with stress, depression, and a desire to lose weight (Kandel 1998; Drug Strategies 1998).

Women are viewed as harder to treat than men. While there is no evidence for this—in fact, women do as well as or better than men in addiction treatment—there is a perception by some treatment staff that women are more difficult. This may reflect stereotypes of women as childlike, dependent, and hysterical (Karpman 1956; Walitzer and Connors 1997).

Addicted women have less money than addicted men. They are more often single parents, which results in lower financial resources. Also, women alcoholics are more likely to drop out of treatment due to financial problems than men (Beckman and Amaro 1986).

What About Men?

Because this is a book about women, the information focuses on them. However, you may be interested to know the other side of the picture—how are men with addictions different? Men have higher rates of addiction, and are more likely to be violent and engage in criminal activity in connection with substance use (Kessler et al. 1994; Wilsnack and Wilsnack 1997). Men are more likely to have legal problems from drinking. They fight and get arrested more and, because they drink more often in public places, they are more likely to be noticed by the police. They have more problems with peers (Tarter, Kirisci, and Mezzich 1997), and have a higher rate of "externalizing disorders" (emotional problems that they direct outward at others), such as antisocial personality (Cottler 1998). They also do more binge drinking (Drug Strategies 1998).

Some History

Many current patterns have existed for a long time. Moreover, societal attitudes have often gone to extremes, playing down and even encouraging substance use in women at some points and at other times expressing excessive alarm at it. It has been observed that, in advertising, "images of glamour and degradation often exist side by side" (Blume 1997a, 485).

✦ Throughout history, there were separate drinking rules for men and women. Ancient Roman law made any use of alcohol by women illegal, and records show several cases where women were put to death for drinking. Drinking is generally considered a sign of full citizenship, and limiting women's use may have been a way to "keep women in their place" (Heath 1993).

✦ Western thought dating back to the ancient Talmud held that alcohol would lead women to promiscuity—the classic "fallen woman." More recently, from 1936 to 1958 the U.S. Distilled Spirits Council had rules prohibiting the use of women in ads for alcoholic beverages (Blume 1997a).

✦ In the nineteenth century, women were the *majority* of drug users, and this included opiate addicts. Women were overmedicated by doctors at a much higher rate than men, often with tinctures, gums, and powders. According to Kandall, "The overmedication of women compared with men has been an issue for the past 150 years, beginning with the image of the Victorian woman as less able to bear pain than a man and therefore more in need of medication. The typical drug addict during this period was a white, upper class woman from the South" (1998, 9-10). Women were commonly prescribed opiates for gynecologic problems and physical and mental exhaustion. Opiates were often the only treatment for many medical problems. Marijuana was commonly prescribed for labor pains, postpartum psychosis, headaches, and gonorrhea (Blume 1997a).

✦ In the early 1900s, women continued to have high rates of addiction. Cocaine and opiates, and many tonics containing these, were legal (Kandall 1998). Indeed, the soda name "Coca-Cola" refers to the cocaine that was part of the recipe for thirty years, until its replacement by caffeine in 1906. Cocaine was believed to be a treatment for opiate and alcohol addiction, and both cocaine and opiates were prescribed for medical problems in children.

✦ In the 1960s and 1970s women in the U.S. tended to abuse prescription drugs, such as amphetamines ("diet pills"), tranquilizers, and alcohol. Advertising touted "happy pills," "miracle drugs," and "peace-of-mind" drugs. By 1967, more than two-thirds of psychoactive prescriptions were for women. Hidden addiction in housewives was common. Kandall concluded that "drug manufacturers have promoted images that portray women as weak and have marketed drugs to women to make a profit" (1998, 14). Increasingly sophisticated strategies were developed to market substances to women, including wine coolers and "women's" brands of cigarettes (Kandall 1998; Kilbourne 2002). In

1966, Odyssey House in New York began as one of the first treatment programs for pregnant women and their children.

✦ In the 1980s, the crack cocaine epidemic focused attention on women as the drug hooked them in record numbers. Thousands of babies were born addicted to crack and underweight, creating a major burden for hospitals and schools. Crack was associated with crime and destroyed neighborhoods. In the late 1980s, federal drug policy began to focus on women as a distinct group, and initiatives were developed to help them and their children (Drug Strategies 1998).

✦ In the 1990s, women's health began to receive greater attention in science and the media for the first time. The need to include women in research studies, to provide better access to health care, and to focus on gender differences in treatment was recognized (Blumenthal 1998).

You Are Not Alone: Rates of Addiction in Women

Overall, women have a lower rate of addiction than men, and this holds true across countries (Fillmore et al. 1997). Recently, however, there has been *convergence*, meaning that among young people the addiction rates of females and males have become almost equivalent. Moreover, the rate of addiction across genders has increased dramatically in the past forty years (Nelson, Heath, and Kessler 1998). While casual use of some drugs has declined (e.g., marijuana and cocaine), addictive use of these drugs has increased (Drug Strategies 1998). Also, heroin, methamphetamine, and new drugs such as oxycontin have become popular. Many drugs are widely available (SAMHSA 2001b). Thus, more people are struggling with addiction problems than in previous generations (Grant 1997). This increase has occurred despite the fact that the overall health of the population has improved in other areas, such as life expectancy, infant survival, medical care, and lowered cholesterol and hypertension (NCHS 2001).

Women and girls in particular are becoming addicted at greater rates than ever before. This includes drinking (including binge drinking), smoking, and abuse of prescription drugs and all types of illegal drugs. Thirty-one million women in the U.S. are estimated to have substance addiction (Drug Strategies 1998). If one includes addictions that are not widely measured, such as gambling, Internet, sex, shopping, exercise, and food, the rates are even higher.

You may be interested to read the following facts:

✦ 18 percent of women in the U.S. develop substance use disorder at some point in their lives; for men the rate is 35 percent. This means that on average across genders, more than one-quarter of the entire population (26 percent) will struggle with addiction to a substance (Kessler et al. 1994). You are indeed not alone!

✦ Substance addiction is the most common psychiatric disorder in the U.S. (Kessler et al. 1994).

+ Women represent about 30 percent of illegal-drug abusers; if prescription drugs were included, the rate would be much higher (Kandall 1998).

+ Women are just as likely as men to use a drug if given the opportunity (NIDA 2000).

+ Women are more likely to become addicted to alcohol than to drugs (Kessler et al. 1994).

+ Among females, young women from fifteen to twenty-four years old have the highest rate of current substance use disorder (Kessler et al. 1994).

+ More than twice as many people have alcohol addiction as drug addiction (Kessler et al. 1994).

+ White women drink more than African-American, Hispanic, or Asian women (Gomberg 1997).

+ Many women drink, but only a small percentage become addicted. For example, 64 percent of women have at least one drink per year, but only 6 percent become addicted. Twenty-five percent of women have alcohol at least once per week (Walitzer and Connors 1997).

+ 23 percent of women are heavy smokers, and 25 percent of women under age twenty-five smoke (Blumenthal 1998).

Society and Addictions

As you can see, if you have a problem, you're not the only one. The rate of addictions has increased dramatically since the 1950s. Indeed, despite over 30 billion dollars spent in the past twenty years toward fighting foreign drug supplies, drugs are cheaper and more widespread than ever (Drug Strategies 1998). Addiction is part of a larger social fabric. The question thus becomes, Why are people—and women in particular—turning to substances more and more as a way to feel better? While there's no one answer, various forces are likely explanations.

Increased stress, especially for women. Women's role used to be solely in the home. Now that most women (60 percent) work outside the home (Drug Strategies 1998), they have more responsibility than ever before. Even when women have the same number of hours on the job as men, they have more household responsibilities and are seen as the primary caretakers of children. Women are still paid less than men for the same work, which can lead to financial stress.

Less community support. The bonds of extended families and communities have been weakened by greater mobility than ever before. Moves and job changes are common. Alienation and loneliness can result, and substances may feel like a solution. Even the health care system has become more fragmented and bureaucratic. You may find yourself shuttled between programs with little sense that anyone really knows you. This is an obstacle to recovery from addiction.

Increased access to addictive activities. Substances never before available are now widespread (e.g., "club drugs" such as ecstasy among young women and various prescription drugs among older women). Activities that used to be for men only, such as drinking in bars, gambling, and casual sex, are now fully available to women.

Less money spent on addiction treatment. Despite the increase in addiction, there is actually less government money being spent on women's addiction treatment than in the early 1980s (Drug Strategies 1998). Long waiting lists and short treatments are common. Even pregnant substance-abusing women, who are one of the most important groups due to the immediate danger to their unborn children, do not have access to enough care. Indeed, only 12 percent of pregnant women needing addiction treatment receive it (Blume 1998).

Greater focus on appearance and success. With the enormous expansion of the media in the past half-century, personal image has become more important. The constant barrage of images can be influential—particularly for women, whose worth is often measured by physical attractiveness (Kilbourne 2002). Many women use substances to lose weight, maintain energy, be more sexual, and fit in socially. The pressure to succeed at work (formerly just a "man's problem") may lead to workaholism and the use of substances as a way to relax.

Society has advanced in many positive ways, giving women more independence, financial success, and options than ever before. Most women would not want to return to the restrictions of former times. But adapting to this high degree of social change can take a toll, making women more vulnerable to addiction. Learning to stay healthy amid all the pressure is key. The need for advocacy—helping women obtain more and better services—is also clear. Thus, it may help to know that whatever you may have done in your life, society too is part of the equation.

Noticing Your Feelings

How do you feel after reading this information? It may be good to check in with yourself. Being aware of feelings is a big part of the recovery process. All feelings are valid; none are bad or wrong. For example, it may be upsetting to read this information, but your reactions can energize you toward healing. Do you feel:

+ **Angry?** Use your anger to help yourself and other women obtain the help that's needed.

+ **Sad?** See your sadness as reflecting important truths. Nonetheless, know that much can be done to improve things.

+ **Worried?** View your worry as a natural reaction to hearing difficult information. Before any real progress occurs, worry is usually present.

+ **Hopeless?** Know that despite the many issues faced by women with addiction, the situation is definitely *not* hopeless. If you keep reading, you'll find many reasons for hope, both for you and for other women.

In short, while women's addictions are indeed a serious and growing problem, within each woman there is always the capacity to shift course, change, and heal.

Who Are the Women with Addiction?

Women's and men's differences in addiction are not the whole story, however. Women also differ greatly among themselves and come from an array of backgrounds. Some represent "invisible" groups outside the mainstream, while others are highly valued in society. If you want, identify any categories that apply to you.

☐ **High-Functioning or High-Status Women.** These women may be wealthy, have celebrity status, or have succeeded professionally in competitive fields such as law, business, or medicine. Their addiction problems may go unnoticed for a long time, as substance abuse may be part of their cultural world—the "blue blood" woman drinking before dinner, the lawyer entertaining clients, or the singer partying on tour. They also may have other addictions, commonly workaholism (which reinforces their financial and work success) and other compulsive activities that create a sense of control, such as eating disorders, exercise, or shopping. The social prominence of such women may mean they have a lot to lose if their addiction became known. In the past two decades, it has become more acceptable for women (such as Kitty Dukakis, Betty Ford, and Drew Barrymore) to talk openly about their problems, but nonetheless it remains difficult. Drinking alone is most common among women who are married, employed, and of upper socioeconomic status. Yet, such women are the *least* likely to be identified as addicted by families and medical staff until the disease is in an advanced stage (Blume 1997b).

☐ **Lesbian / Bisexual / Transgender Women.** LGBT (lesbian, gay, bisexual, transgender) individuals are "more likely to use alcohol and drugs, have higher rates of substance abuse, are less likely to abstain from use, and are more likely to continue heavy drinking into later life" (SAMHSA 2001a, xiii). Studies that have compared them with heterosexuals have found that 20 to 25 percent are heavy alcohol users compared to 3 to 10 percent of the heterosexuals studied (SAMHSA 2001a). They also appear to use more party drugs, such as ecstasy and ketamine ("special K"). Gay bars have historically been the place for much socializing among lesbians. This bar culture, and the homophobia that oppresses lesbians, are believed to result in an increased rate of alcoholism. Indeed, one-third of lesbians are estimated to be alcoholic. Substances may also be used to cope with keeping one's sexual orientation secret, exclusion from mainstream society, and the stress of violence against gays and lesbians. The lesbian community may also be reluctant to deal openly with addiction because society already stigmatizes them for their sexual orientation. Some fear engaging in treatment due to the history of insensitivity and homophobia in the medical community (Plumb 1998; SAMHSA 2001a).

☐ **Women with Medical Illness or Disability.** Substances are often used to lessen physical pain associated with cancer, AIDS, chronic pain, head injury, or other medical problems. The tendency to become addicted to painkillers or use nonprescribed "medication" (such as alcohol) is well known. Indeed, the rate of addiction among the physically ill may be twice that of the general population (Chapman 1998). Women use medical services at a higher rate than men and receive more prescribed psychoactive medication than men (Kandall 1998); their potential for addiction is thus high. Addiction may also lead to a wide variety of physical injuries and illnesses, including sexually transmitted diseases, head injury (e.g., due to drunk driving), hepatitis, and HIV. The lifestyle of addiction also commonly leads to the neglect of medical care and health behaviors.

☐ **Teenage Girls.** Drinking, substance use, and smoking among teen girls is growing at a rate never seen before. Use of most substances increased among teen girls in the 1990s, including marijuana, nicotine, inhalants, cocaine, stimulants, LSD, and prescription drugs. Some substances, such as marijuana, saw a huge increase, more than doubling. It used to be that teen girls used much less than teen boys, but now they are basically equivalent (Drug Strategies 1998). Indeed, drinking and smoking are increasing much faster for teen girls than boys, and there is less social disapproval of girls' binge drinking than ever before. Teens who engage in substance use often have other behavior problems, such as early pregnancy, delinquency, and truancy (Drug Strategies 1998). Teen girls who develop addiction have lower achievement, less responsibility, and less control over their feelings (e.g., anger and impulsivity) (Brook 1998). Studies of chronic substance-abusing women show identifiable behavior patterns in adolescence; thus, it's important to identify addiction early (Schnoll 1998). A developmental challenge for all girls is the tendency during the early teen years to place too much emphasis on their looks and ability to please others rather than on their own interests. This is also typically the first time they're exposed to substance use and other risky behaviors, making it a highly vulnerable period.

☐ **Women in the Helping Professions.** The tendency to "give all" and lose touch with one's own needs is a known danger in the helping professions. Substance addiction is in fact the "single most frequent disabling illness for the medical professional," although actual rates of addiction are not higher than among the general population (Gallegos and Talbott 1997, 745). Access to prescription medication (for doctors), long work hours, stress from changes in the health care system, and isolated work may be associated with a variety of addictions, including substance abuse, workaholism, and overeating. Women may be at particular risk, as taking care of others is their traditional family role, which may be heightened by a work role as a helper as well.

☐ **Older Women.** Women live an average of seven years longer than men, and since 1900 women's life expectancy has increased by about thirty years (Blumenthal 1998). As they grow older, more women than men become drug dependent (Kandel 1998). Although older women are only 11 percent of the population, they receive 25 percent of prescriptions—2.5 times as many as older men. Also, mixing medications (*polypharmacy*) is high among older women (Blumenthal 1998). One large study of the elderly, found that men drink to pass the time while women drink to reduce depression (Graham and Braun 1999). One of the most common patterns among women is the use of substances to cope with aging and "lost roles" throughout the lifespan: widowhood, the empty nest as children leave home, divorce, and retirement (Blume 1997b). The isolation of older women due to retirement, inability to drive, and living alone may make it difficult for them to access care (CSAT 1994a).

☐ **Minority Women.** A common belief is that minorities use substances more than whites. Yet many groups of minority women (African-American, Hispanic, Asian) have lower rates of use and abuse than Caucasian women (Gomberg 1997). Some populations, however, such as American Indians, have much higher rates (Jumper-Thurman 1998). One pattern seen in immigrants is the tendency for addiction to rise in later generations as they adapt to American culture (Sanders-Phillips 1998). Aside from numbers, minorities face greater hurdles in obtaining help with addiction, including lower identification of addiction, less access to care, greater punishment for addiction (e.g., courts are more likely to sentence minorities for substance-related infractions than Caucasians), racism, and lack of culturally sensitive treatments (Kandall 1998; Rhodes and Johnson 1997). Indeed, while African-American women drink less than Caucasian women, they are twice as likely to die from alcoholism (McCrady and Raytek 1993).

☐ **Rural Women.** Although rates of addiction are not higher in rural than in urban areas (Kessler et al. 1994), addiction treatment is much more difficult to obtain. The lack of specialized services, the more traditional roles of women, and the increased stigma of addiction in small communities may make it especially hard for women to seek care. A sense of isolation among rural women with addictions is common (Boyd and Hauenstein 1997).

☐ **Single Professional Women.** Single women are among the most likely to be heavy drinkers (Gomberg 1997). They also report frequent use of alcohol as an escape from the demands of their jobs (Blum and Roman 1997). Keeping up with both work and home life, particularly for single working mothers with children, is associated with more drinking (Blum and Roman 1997). Opportunities for women to use substances are increased in male-dominated professions.

☐ **Pregnant Women.** Despite national ad campaigns in bars and liquor stores, drinking among pregnant women increased "dramatically" in the past decade (Drug Strategies 1998). From 1992 to 1995, the number who consumed any alcohol rose 60 percent and the number who drank frequently (at least seven drinks a week) increased fourfold. Of the 4 million women who give birth each year, one in eight uses alcohol, tobacco, or other drugs during the week before delivery; rates are higher among whites than minority women. Children whose mothers smoked or drank during pregnancy have higher rates of many medical problems, including neurological and respiratory problems, seizures, sudden infant death, and learning disorders. Stillbirths, miscarriages, and premature births are also increased. The longer a pregnant woman drinks during pregnancy, the lower the child's mental capacity. Even becoming abstinent in the third trimeseter can improve outcomes. Women who smoke or use drugs during pregnancy are more likely to have children who eventually smoke or use drugs. Unfortunately, treatment programs for pregnant women are rare. While there is often tremendous social judgment of pregnant women who abuse substances, there is extremely little care available to them. This is particularly true for women who are poor: one recent survey of public child welfare agencies across the country found that they were able to find treatment for only 20 percent of pregnant women addicts (Drug Strategies 1998). The guilt and self-blame among pregnant women for harming their children can last a lifetime, yet often they are unable to get help when they need it. Criminal prosecution of pregnant women who use substances has been widely condemned by the medical field. It prevents women from seeking help for addiction and prenatal care during pregnancy and ultimately increases harm to the unborn child (Blume 1997a; Paltrow 1998).

☐ **College Women.** In 1997, 40 percent of college women reported binge drinking (four drinks in a row) during the previous two weeks. Social norms that used to deter women from binge drinking are disappearing; there is less disapproval and perception of risk. In sororities and fraternities binge drinking is even more common, with four out of five residents reporting binge drinking. College drinking is involved in two-thirds of unsafe sexual practices (e.g., not using a condom) and three-quarters of all date rapes (Drug Strategies 1998). Other addictions, such as binge eating, compulsive exercise, and workaholism, may also be particular risks for college women.

☐ **Women in Prison.** Substance abuse is the main reason women enter prison, and is the single most common health problem of women there (Henderson 1998). In the past twenty years, the number of women prisoners has soared and women have become the fastest growing group, largely due to drug-related offenses (Mullings 1998). Sadly, women prisoners are mostly young, uneducated, poor, and minority. They have worse mental and physical health than women outside prison. Compared to addicted men in prison, addicted women have lower incomes, more employment problems, and higher rates of physical and sexual abuse, suicidal behavior, depression, and anxiety (Peters et al. 1997). They are more likely to be nonviolent with no prior criminal history and no high-level drug trafficking; often they are involved in drug crimes through spouses or boyfriends (Battle et al., in press). Tragically, the majority of women behind bars leave children under age eighteen at home, and their children are at increased risk of substance abuse (Drug Strategies 1998). In short, "drugs are the common denominator for women and girls in the criminal justice system" (Drug Strategies 1998, 23).

Other populations at risk of addiction include:

☐ **Housewives**

☐ **Inner city women**

☐ **Women veterans**

☐ **Women with emotional disorders**

☐ **Women with a history of violence or trauma**

As these groups demonstrate, it is important to recognize that while female gender plays a role in addictions, so do other characteristics. We're all subject to the "luck of the draw" in life—factors such as medical and emotional problems, geography, age, race, and family history—that can shape addiction.

It is a step in self-awareness to recognize that while ultimately one must take responsibility for one's choices in life (such as the abuse of alcohol and drugs), there are also contexts that make people vulnerable to addiction. For example, a woman may begin using substances to block memories of childhood sexual abuse. She may be addicted for many years and have enormous self-blame by the time she receives help—even though the child abuse and lack of help were not her fault. The rest of this book is devoted to helping you explore your own identity and take action to improve your life. Tomorrow can be different.

One Woman's Story

The following story is from a woman who achieved thirty years of sobriety from substances. She went from being an incest survivor, battered woman, and severe polysubstance addict to becoming a social worker who now helps others in their recovery. She attributes her success to a combination of 12-step work and therapy. She gives this story in the hope that it might help someone else. After you read it, you may want to tell your own story, and some suggestions will be offered to guide you in that.

I started drinking at the age of fifteen, usually with people who were older than me. At that time I looked and acted older than fifteen. I got caught up with a crowd of pretty heavy drinkers. We would drink in sandpits and cemeteries, as young people sometimes do, and by sixteen I was in bars with false IDs. At seventeen, I was a daily drinker. I left home when I was seventeen and lived in rooming houses. At one time I was homeless for about six months. I had various odd jobs. I graduated eighth in my high school class, but the drinking took me to jobs that were "less than." I started off with a good job after high school but was asked to leave because of my drinking. So I got a series of low-level jobs; I would drink on the job and no one would really notice.

When I was eighteen I met someone in a bar and married him two weeks later in a blackout. I don't remember getting married, but there was a piece of paper proving that I had. I didn't know this person, but he was a substance abuser and I soon began to see that he was also a batterer. I became a battered wife. I drank a lot in those days to cover up the pain of the mistakes I had made. I grew up in a home where if you made mistakes you lived with them, and I figured that I had made this mistake so I had to live with it—it was my punishment in life. I stayed with him for eleven years. Before that I had been very outgoing and had resisted every kind of verbal or physical assault, but with him I was reduced to coping by drinking.

After the first year of marriage I ended up addicted to prescription drugs and later to street drugs because I couldn't get enough prescriptions. I was taking anything and everything and I didn't know half the time what I was taking. I mixed it all with alcohol—I had many close calls with death, and at the time I would have welcomed it. It was my aim in life not to live through another day of drinking. This was even at the expense of my children. I had six children through this marriage, and though I loved my children a great deal, I could not cope with my marriage and the poverty. I lived in a great deal of poverty—half of the time I didn't have any lights or heat, but I had these children. Eventually I started filing charges of assault and battery against my husband, with the intention of going through with them regardless of the consequences. Unfortunately, the courts at the time didn't listen to most battered women because they thought they wouldn't follow through. So at the end of this eleven-year period I had filed fourteen charges of assault and battery that the court had never processed.

After eleven years I sought a divorce. I continued to drink very heavily and on one of my last drinking bouts I ended up being pronounced dead on arrival at the hospital. I was revived by a heart doctor. I was introduced to Al-Anon by a social worker at the hospital. I didn't know what it was—I had never heard of Alcoholics Anonymous or Al-Anon. I didn't even know anybody who drank like I did. I came from a small town and lived in a neighborhood where if someone had a couple of drinks, that was unusual. No one really drank. My father was a social drinker—he could have one drink this year and not have another for ten years. My family was dysfunctional in other ways, but drinking wasn't one of them. I went to the Al-Anon meeting and it sparked something that I thought was long dead—the glimmer of hope that there might be some way I could get out of this mess. Al-Anon was very beneficial to me; three years into it, it helped me understand that I didn't deserve the punishment. Regardless of the drinking, I didn't deserve to be battered.

I filed for divorce behind my husband's back, and when he found out about it he became extremely assaultive, breaking into my house on a weekly basis. Fortunately for me I had managed to get into a 12-step program for my drinking. I realized that I had a significant problem with alcohol and drugs. It ceased to matter to me whether or not he killed me—it would have been okay because I wasn't going to live like that anymore and I wasn't going to drink and drug over it. I went into the 12-step program in April and my husband was dead by August of that year. He died as violently as he had lived—he shot up a barroom. Just a week prior to his death he'd threatened me and my six children. We were living in a housing project at the time, with a lot of elderly people; if he'd come there, a lot of them besides me would have been either dead or hurt. After he died I was still very shell-shocked with fear; I thought he was still there. People kept telling me that I couldn't stay sober in fear. To that point, I had only managed to put six months of sobriety together before I had a relapse. I went into a blackout sober—I didn't even remember picking up a drink. I had become extremely overwrought and couldn't remember where I was or where I was going. That led me back to AA. From that time until now, I have thirty years clean. A lot of things have changed.

Things did not go well for me in the first five years of my recovery. I had a lot of family problems that had to be taken care of, a lot of issues with my children that had to be dealt with. But the one thing I did understand was that drinking or drugging would not make it any better. For me, staying away from a drink or drug for a day was an accomplishment. That was success. I was in my twenties when I got sober, and feel like my whole life really turned around. I managed somehow to do most of the 12-step program. I'm still involved in recovery. But I really struggled with the spiritual part of the program in the beginning. I equated spirituality with religion, but eventually realized that it had more to do with my relationship with myself, with my friends, with my community, and with the world. That made more sense to me. If it wasn't for the spiritual part of the program I probably wouldn't have had thirty years sober.

I can't say that it was easy. It wasn't easy. It wasn't easy raising six kids with just a high school education, but I managed to put one foot in front of the other, managed to get some very good accounting jobs. I just kept showing up and doing all the right things that needed to be done and taking courses here and there. I also met another man and dated him for five years, and we've been married fourteen years now. We have a very different marriage than my first one. He's a good man and a good provider, and there's no battering. I decided I'd go back to school, so I worked part-time and put myself through four years of college in psychology.

Then I went to work with substance abusers, which is my favorite thing. For me it's about "passing it on." And especially for women—women struggle so, in early recovery, just like I did. Women have to do recovery different from men. I don't mean that to sound sexist, it's just that it's different— women are usually single parents, and there's a lot of shame and guilt. I had a lot of that around my own children. I never hit my children, but I was not emotionally available to them. Today I am; today I'm a good mother. I was very fortunate that I got sober early enough that my children and grandchildren have a mother and a grandmother who's there all the time, both physically and emotionally. I think it's a great accomplishment that my kids depend on me to be there and that, at the same time, I see their independence as individuals. They're wonderful people and I'm really proud that they're my children. I've also done a lot of community work: I worked in a prison for over ten years, and I did a lot of work with adolescents and substance abuse. In 1997 I went back to earn my master's degree in social work.

I feel that this is what sobriety is—sobriety means that you turn to a life that gives you dignity and self-respect. When I first got sober I was best friends with my shoes because I couldn't look people in the eye. I couldn't face the world outside. I felt so bad about what I had done and what I had become. It feels good to keep my head up and to know that sobriety offers dignity along with a clear head. I can accomplish the things I used to just sit there and think about. I realize that colors are bright, and not gray and black—I thought things were gray and black when I was first in recovery.

It takes a lot of stick-to-it. You know, you have to just keep putting one foot in front of the other. For me, "one day at a time" was a very hard concept to get. But I had to learn to keep my recovery in the day, and I still do that. Even though I have almost thirty years, I don't want to forget that I'm only "that far" away from a drink and a drug. I don't want to forget because then I'll forget what it was like to be back there—the pain I felt, the emotional and physical withdrawal. I did it before detoxes were fully available, so I did it all at a 12-step program. I shook in those meetings. I felt so keyed up that if someone dropped something I'd go through the ceiling. What I have today I just don't want to give up, so I need to remember what I went through to get here.

It was all definitely worth the struggle. I wouldn't even change the fact of my drinking and drugging, even though it was horrific. I mean, a lot of things happened that came out of all that. It's so worth the struggle to keep myself clean and sober. You don't get dignity by drinking, and as a woman, I value and cherish my dignity—as a person and as a human being too, but also as a woman who has character.

Recovery is different for women. For example, I was an incest victim. I received a lot of help around that but in the beginning the 12 steps were presented as "making amends," and I found myself making amends inappropriately—to people who should have been making amends to me. I found that I had to rework the 12 steps. For me, recovery was a combination of the 12-step program and therapy. Without my therapist I would not have gained what I've gained.

Women's recovery is different because of the amount of shame women have, and because of trying to juggle everything. There's a tremendous amount of shame inside most women about their substance abuse. Society—no matter how far we've come with the knowledge of addiction—still does not see a woman who's drunk or abusing pills or stoned the way they see a man. They always go after the woman for being a bad mother. So women bear the brunt, even in recovery, even when they're trying to get better. I'm not saying anything bad about the 12 steps, but sometimes they have to be redesigned. I may need to do something different than my male counterparts.

Telling Your Story

Now it's time to tell your story, if you choose to. It is always up to you whether to try the exercises in this book, but you may find them helpful.

1. **Find a way to tell your story.** This might be writing, talking into a tape recorder or video camera, or creating an art project such as a collage or drawing. Pick the way that you like best. If you want, use a favorite color pen and some beautiful paper to honor your story.

2. **Tell the story of your addiction,** noting the following points:

   ✦ **No putting yourself down**. Your story needs to be respectful of what you lived through. There were reasons life went the way it did. This doesn't mean things went smoothly, and it also doesn't mean you did everything right (no one does!). It just means your story should reflect the deepest understanding you have about yourself, without harsh blame.

✦ **If you have a history of trauma or violence, do not provide details about that now.** This might include child abuse, rape, or domestic violence. While these may be very important parts of your life and highly connected to your addiction, it may not be safe to talk about them yet. Early in recovery you need to be self-protective, taking on only as much as you can handle. Trauma is known to be upsetting, and you may be surprised by how much feeling will emerge if you describe it. Some people find their addiction gets worse or they become suicidal. For now, either leave it out or just mention it in a few words without going into details. Once you're further along, you can tell your story again more fully. See chapter 3 for more on this topic.

✦ **Include good as well as bad.** Even if you're early in recovery, notice what you've done right. Perhaps you reached out for help at points, made it through some tough times, or had positive moments along the way. No matter how awful, there were ways you got through it—notice these good sides too.

3. **Decide whether you want anyone to hear your story.** You could go to a self-help group and read it there, take it to your therapist, or tell it to a close friend or partner. Or you can just keep it for yourself.

4. **Listen for themes.** Many people find insights as they tell their story. Listen for discoveries—a new understanding of why you did what you did, or a sense of compassion for how hard it's been.

_____

_____

_____

_____

_____

How This Book Was Developed

This book is based on my work with women who have been addicted. When I began in the field in 1992, I was drawn to helping addicted women who had a history of trauma, typically childhood abuse. As I learned more about these women through treating them, hearing their stories, and working with front-line clinicians, I came to understand how often they had been thwarted in their attempts to get help. Their trauma issues often went unrecognized, their need for both mental health and addiction treatment was often not met, and their need to connect with other women was hindered by an absence of gender-based services. At times, I heard statements that were stunning in their ignorance of women's experience. "I don't believe in trauma," said one treater. "A certain number will kill themselves, and there's nothing we can do about it," said another. I also heard many very moving stories of women who obtained help from caring providers. This contrast between the worst and the best in the treatment field made me aware of the need for much more support for women in their recovery.

During my work, I've also been privileged to get to know some of the original leaders in the field of women's addiction treatment from the 1970s, including Vivian Brown, Stephanie Covington, Margaret Cramer, Norma Finkelstein, Beth Glover Reed, and Joan Zweben. They were highly supportive and helped me understand new dimensions of women's treatment.

We are all more human than otherwise, it has been said, and my work with addicted men has been just as gratifying as my work with women. In my career, I have benefited from men and women mentors, and have seen men suffer their own difficulties in trying to get help for recovery. Thus, I hope this workbook will be viewed not simply as one for women per se, but as one that underscores the idea that effective help is based on truly hearing people's needs and experiences. The spotlight here is on women, but the need for validation and understanding is universal.

☎ Resources

Would you like to understand more? The following free resources can help you with the key topics of this chapter: women, addiction, special populations, and addiction health issues. At the end of later chapters, resources will be provided on other topics.

Women

National Women's Health Information Center Provides information, regional events, research, etc.	800-994-WOMAN	www.4woman.gov
Healthfinder To locate reliable health information on the Web	[no website]	www.healthfinder.gov
National Health Information Center Government information center about health issues	800-336-4797	www.health.gov/nhic

Addiction

National Drug Information, Treatment, and Referral Line Confidential resource for obtaining assistance by the Center for Substance Abuse Treatment	800-662-HELP	www.drughelp.org
National Clearinghouse for Alcohol and Drug Information Resources for addiction recovery, including videos, pamphlets, monographs, and research reports	800-729-6686	www.health.org
Office on Smoking and Health	800-CDC-1311	www.cdc.gov
National Institute on Drug Abuse Note: their Info Fax Service provides information that can be faxed to you	888-NIH-NIDA	www.nida.nih.gov
National Institute on Alcohol Abuse and Alcoholism	[no 800 number]	www.niaaa.nih.gov
Alcohol and Drug Healthline	800-821-4357	www.samhsa.gov
American Council for Drug Education	800-488-DRUG	www.acde.org

| American Council on Alcoholism | 800-527-5344 | www.recovery2000.com |

Note: See chapter 2 for self-help resources (e.g., AA).

Special Populations

Office of Minority Health Resource Center	800-444-6472	www.omhrc.gov
National Latina Health Organization	510-534-1362	latino.sscnet.ucla.edu/ women/nlho/
National Black Women's Health Project	202-543-9311	www.nbwhp.org
National Asian Women's Health Organization	415-989-9747	www.nawho.org
Native American Women's Health Education Resource Center	605-487-7072	www.nativeshop.org
Caribbean Women's Health Association	718-826-2942	www.aidsnyc/cwha

Addiction Health Issues

Hepatitis Hotline	800-223-0719	www.cdc.gov/ncidod/ diseases/hepatitis
Hepatitis Foundation International	800-891-0707	www.hepfi.org
HIV/AIDS Treatment Information Service	800-448-0440	www.hivatis.org
CDC National AIDS Hotline	800-342-AIDS (English) 800-344-7432 (Spanish)	www.cdc.gov/hw/ hivinfo/nah.htm
CDC National AIDS Clearinghouse	800-458-5231 (English) 800-243-7012 (Spanish)	www.cdcnpin.org/ pubs/start.htm
National Center for Injury Prevention and Control	770-488-1506	www.cdc.gov/ncipc

| Centers for Disease Control and Prevention—National Immunization Program
Vaccines and referrals for hepatitis, flu, and other illnesses | 800-232-2522 (English)
800-232-0233 (Spanish) | www.cdc.gov/nip |

CHAPTER 2

Understanding
Addiction

This chapter will help you explore whether you have an addiction problem and, if so, to select a model of recovery. The term "understanding" in the title is meant in two senses—obtaining new knowledge, and also taking a compassionate view toward yourself and your addiction. As Molly Goode (1999) says, "Your heart whispers, so listen closely."

People can get addicted to just about anything: mountain climbing, collecting antiques, a person, a substance, gambling, chocolate, exercise, TV, sex, or spending money. But it's not the thing itself that is the problem. It's the compulsion to keep doing it excessively or recklessly that is the problem. One drink is fine; it's when it becomes seven drinks and a citation for "driving under the influence" that it's a problem. Going shopping is fun; it's when it leads you into debt and destroys your family that it is a problem.

Addiction also doesn't mean just "physical dependence." That's an old definition that's not entirely accurate (Volpicelli et al. 2001). For example, some highly addictive substances, such as cocaine and methamphetamine, do not cause physical withdrawal symptoms if a person stops using them, which is the definition of physical dependence (Margolis and Zweben 1998). Addictions that do not involve mind-altering substances, such as food, gambling, sex, and shopping, may also have no physical withdrawal symptoms, but have been found parallel to substance addictions in other important ways (Glick and Halperin 1997; Gold, Johnson, and Stennie 1997; Goodman 1997; Shaffer 1997).

Ultimately, it's up to you to decide whether your behavior has taken a turn for the worse or whether it's under control. The goal of this chapter is to help you make that evaluation. Know too that there is no judgment involved: this is about you and how you want to live your life. It's peering into your soul to better understand what's really going on. It's not about labels, finger-wagging, or blame. And it's not about who you are as a person. Terrific, good people get addicted all the time due to various factors—genetic vulnerability, family history, who they happen to become friends with, where they grew up, and so on. Addiction is never about your essential worth as a person. But it is about quality of life: whether you are living in a way that gives you what life is capable of at it's best, or whether you have sunk to a diminished, addiction-focused existence. Or perhaps you are somewhere in the middle of these extremes, just trying to get a sense of which path you may be on. The key is to evaluate where you are now. Indeed, it's been said that while getting help early is important for anyone with an addiction problem, this may be especially important for women, whose addictions are less likely to be noticed in the early stages than are men's (Walitzer and Connors 1997). So let us proceed.

What Is Addiction?

Addiction is "the compulsion to use despite negative consequences" (Leshner 1999). This means that you keep using over and over, no matter what it's doing to your life. It may feel as though you're watching yourself self-destruct but can't stop, as in a bad dream.

One description of women addicted to gambling conveys this sense of desperate repetition: "These women escaped sad emotions in a noisy gambling environment—a self-destructive environment of non-reality.... [They] found themselves out of control, helpless to pay off debt, thinking illogically about losing money and thinking illogically about solutions. Their only solution for paying off debt was to try harder, and to try harder meant gambling more" (Rich 1998, 6823).

While people may vary in their type of addiction—substances, food, exercise, Internet, gambling, sex, shopping—addiction itself has a common set of characteristics. Some people have a few characteristics, while others have them all. Some people have one addiction, while others have several. Some have mild versions, while others' addictions are severe. In the next section, you'll have the opportunity to explore your level of addiction. Later we'll explore ways you can help yourself if you do have a problem. There are many ways to heal from an addiction if you have one and, for a subset of people, it may not mean giving up the addictive activity. So as you go through the questions, just be as honest as you can without being too concerned about where it all leads. One truth you'll discover is that honesty with yourself will always lead to something good over time.

Listening to Yourself

Would you like to take a look at your own life? If so, answer the following questions. They represent the standard definition in the field of an addiction (APA 1994). Know that you can keep your answers private, or you can share them with a trusted person in your life (e.g., a therapist, family member, or friend). You can also copy the pages and have that person fill it out about you to give you feedback. For addiction, feedback is known to be especially helpful, as others may have a perspective that can create a more complete picture. Remember, no matter what you find out, having the courage to explore these issues is a truly positive step.

Part 1: What addiction(s) may be a problem for you? Check off all that you're wondering about. Note: for all drugs that could be prescribed, check them off only if the drug is taken not as prescribed (e.g., without a prescription, more than prescribed, or excessively prescribed—i.e., "doctor shopping" to get multiple prescriptions).

☐ Alcohol

☐ Other Drug

    ☐ Amphetamines (e.g., speed, diet pills)

    ☐ Cannabis (marijuana, hash)

    ☐ Cocaine

    ☐ Hallucinogens (e.g., ecstasy, LSD, mushrooms)

    ☐ Inhalants (e.g., glue, paint, gasoline)

    ☐ Opioids (e.g., heroin, morphine, methadone)

    ☐ Phenylcyclindine (e.g., PCP, ketamine)

☐ Sedatives (e.g., sleeping pills, tranquilizers)

☐ Polysubstance (at least three of the above groups, with no one drug of choice)

☐ Other drug(s): _____

☐ Nicotine (i.e., smoking)

☐ Gambling

☐ Internet

☐ Food (See also the section on eating disorders in chapter 4.)

☐ Sex

☐ Exercise

☐ A person (e.g., romantic partner whom you obsess about)

☐ TV

☐ Shopping/spending money

☐ Collecting (e.g., antiques)

☐ Work

☐ Relationships (e.g., inability to be alone, sex addiction)

☐ Self-harm (e.g., cutting, burning, self-mutilation)

☐ Plastic surgery

☐ Other: _____

☐ Other: _____

Part 2: For each area you checked off above, ask yourself the questions below. They are drawn from the widely accepted psychiatric definition of substance use disorder (APA 1994). Copy the pages if you want to explore more than one addiction. Later on, we'll interpret your answers, but for now, just notice what's true for you. Keep in mind that the questions were developed for substances, so some questions may not apply to other addictions (e.g., questions 5 and 6). Even among substances, there may be some variation (e.g., question 6 may not apply to some substances).

For each question, fill in the blank line with the addiction you are exploring. For example, if it's cocaine, the first question would be "Do you do <u>cocaine</u> so much that you don't fulfill your obligations?"

Answer all questions for the *past twelve months*. If your behavior varied over the twelve months, take the period of time when it was at its worst. If you don't understand a question, leave it blank for now.

	Yes	No	Maybe
1. Do you do _____ so much that you don't fulfill your obligations? *For example, you show up late for work, don't take good care of your children, or let go of normal tasks (cleaning house, paying bills).*			
2. Do you keep doing _____ in situations that are physically dangerous? *For example, you drink and drive or get high and operate machinery.*			
3. Do you keep doing _____ even though it causes repeated legal problems for you? *For example, you have multiple arrests for drug possession, or spend so much money that creditors are suing you.*			
4. Do you keep doing _____ even though it causes repeated social problems for you? *For example, you have arguments with your partner about your addiction, or get into physical fights when you drink.*			
5. Do you need more _____ to get the same effect? *(tolerance)* *For example, you need three drinks to get the buzz you used to get from one, or you cut yourself more and more severely.*			
6. If you stop doing _____ do you feel bad physically (*withdrawal*, e.g., sweating, nausea, hand tremors, or inability to sleep)? *For example, if you don't drink, you have these problems. Note: Also check "yes" if you drink to avoid experiencing them.*			
7. Do you do _____ in larger amounts or over a longer time than you intended? *For example, you say you'll have just one drink but end up having many or you go shopping "just for an hour" and stay all day.*			
8. Have you tried to stop doing _____ and not been able to? *For example, you tried to quit drinking but keep going back to it, or you tried cutting up your credit cards but keep getting new ones.*			

	Yes	No	Maybe
9. Do you spend a lot of time doing _____ ? *For example, you spend every night at the casino, or your TV watching leaves you no time to see friends.*			
10. Have you given up important activities because of _____ ? *For example, you no longer socialize, play sports, or pursue career advancement.*			
11. Do you keep doing _____ even though it's making a physical or emotional problem worse? *For example, you keep doing cocaine even though it always gets you depressed, or you keep exercising excessively even though you're already injured from it.*			

Part 3: How did you score? Check off any below that fit you.

☐ **Dependence.** For items 5 through 11: How many "yes" answers did you have?_____. If you had three or more, you are considered to have a *dependence problem*. This means that you have a severe addiction to that activity. If you had fewer than three "yes" answers, go to the next question.

☐ **Abuse.** For items 1 through 4: How many "yes" answers did you have?_____. If you had one or more, you are considered to have an *abuse problem*. This means that you have a less severe addiction to that activity, but it's still a problem.

☐ **Possible Problem.** If you said "yes" to some questions, but not enough to meet the definition of either dependence or abuse, or if you said "maybe" to several of the questions, it could mean that you're on your way to developing an addiction, or that you're in the process of working on your addiction (e.g., perhaps you're currently in treatment).

☐ **No Problem.** If you did not answer "yes" or "maybe" to any of the questions, then you would appear to have no problem. Even so, you may want to learn more about addiction.

☐ **Unclear.** You may have had difficulty answering some questions or you may have a mix of responses that makes it difficult to circle one of the categories. That's okay. Read the next section to help you decide.

Negative Impact

Most people say that what helped them see their addiction most clearly was the direct harm to their lives (Fletcher 2001). The five areas in this section are typically impacted by addiction (McLellan et al. 1992). Describe any that you notice in yourself.

Relationship problems. These may include using that results in not being there for your family; people expressing concern about your use; isolating; or spending time with dangerous people. Describe the relationship problems you notice:

_____

_____

_____

_____

Legal problems. These may include using that results in driving under the influence; loss of custody of children; arrest; or illegal behavior. Describe the legal problems you notice.

_____

_____

_____

_____

Physical problems. These may include using that results in unsafe sex; a worsening medical condition such as diabetes or infection; or neglecting your body. Describe the physical problems you notice:

_____

_____

_____

_____

Emotional problems. These may include using that results in depression, anxiety, or anger; "seeing things"; wanting to hurt yourself or others; low self-esteem; guilt; or shame. Describe the emotional problems you notice:

_____

_____

_____

_____

Work problems. These may include using that results in being fired, missing work, or poor performance. Describe the work problems you notice.

_____

_____

_____

_____

Self-Awareness Summary

How concerned are you about your use?

0	1	2	3
Not concerned	A little concerned	Moderately concerned	Extremely concerned

How much of an addiction problem do you feel you have?

0	1	2	3
No problem	A little problem	Moderate problem	Extreme problem

If you answered anything above 0 on either question, you could benefit from exploring more while keeping an open mind.

Sorting It Out When It's Unclear

You may still feel unsure whether or not you have an addiction. Indeed, addictions are known for being hard to evaluate just on your own. Also, the questions in this chapter were developed for substances; other addictions, such as work or sex, may not fit neatly into that framework. You may have found that your answers were different than someone else who filled them out about you (if you chose that option), and thus may feel confused about "who's right."

If you're unclear whether you have an addiction, here are some suggestions.

Seek out a professional opinion. You could set up an appointment at a local substance abuse clinic, community mental health agency, or other resource. (See the resources section at the end of this chapter for ways to locate one in your area.) Be sure to find a professional who has experience treating addiciton. You could also decide to attend a self-help meeting, such as AA, and get feedback from people there. While they are not professionals, they may have a lot of experience to help guide you.

Find out more about addiction. You can keep reading this book even if you're not yet clear whether you have a problem. You can also search the Internet or a local library or bookstore to read more about addiction. You can request free information from the government (see the resources section at the end of chapter 1). In short, the more you understand about addiction from reputable sources, the more you can accurately evaluate your own situation. Often it's a matter of education. Try not to rely on any one source (e.g., what a friend tells you, or what you read from one book); rather, go to as many sources as you can so you can piece together a full picture of what's really going on for you.

Work on it even if you don't have a "label" for it. As they say, labels are great for cans of soup, but not for people. Some people are offended by words such as "addiction," "dependence," or "abuse." Perhaps, for now, just work on whatever you feel is a problem. One of the greatest dangers for women with addiction is waiting too long to get help. If labels get in your way, just focus on the specific problems that led you to picking up this book. You'll do fine if you keep going, and perhaps by the end of the book you'll have a clearer vision of how you see yourself.

More About Addictions

Aside from the "yes/no" approach to addiction, some additional concepts may be helpful. These give a feel for addictions and how they operate. Think of an addiction as a relationship of sorts—your goal is to get to know this part of your life as closely as you can. Underline any ideas that feel relevant to your life.

Addictions May Be Unconscious

If your addiction is unconscious, you may find yourself doing an addictive behavior over and over without knowing why, even if you want to stop. Or you may feel split, with one side wanting to stop and another that persists with the addiction. Also very common is *denial*—believing or pretending there's no problem even though it's clear to the people around you that there is a problem. None of this means you're crazy or mentally ill. It's the nature of addictions to take hold without a person being aware of what's really going on. Some of this is biological, as with alcohol or drugs, where the substance itself can create physical dependence. But for all addictions, at least some part of it is psychological and relates to your innermost feelings and experiences. These may run very deep, and it's common in early recovery to not yet be fully aware of how you ended up at this place. The main strategy is to stay curious about yourself, to view your recovery as a journey where the goal is to understand who you really are. This understanding will emerge over time as you work on your addiction, get feedback from others, and keep learning. But for now, just recognize that these mysteries of the self are part of addiction for everyone. Indeed, recovery can be viewed as "waking up," "becoming aware," or "getting to know yourself."

Addictions Are Often Secret

Most people feel ashamed, guilty, or worried about their addiction and may not feel comfortable telling anyone about it. It may feel as though there's no one safe to tell—that you'll be judged or embarrassed, or that people won't take it seriously. For example, addiction to sex can lead to joking. Addiction to work can sound like it's not a real problem. Addiction to drugs can make you feel like you're weak or a failure. You may have had a bad experience in treatment, where someone didn't understand you when you tried to talk about it. For women in particular, isolation in addiction is common, more so than for men (Blume 1998). As you progress in your recovery, you'll find that it gets easier to figure out who you can trust with your secrets, who can understand them, and who can help you. For now, just know that this secrecy is dangerous—it feeds the addiction because it prevents you from getting support and help. In AA they say, "You're only as sick as you are secret." In chapter 6, we'll talk more about how to open up to others about addiction.

You May Find Yourself Replacing One Addiction With Another

It's a well-known phenomenon that giving up one addiction can lead to substituting another, unless you get support to avoid this pattern. You may give up marijuana and begin drinking more, for example. It doesn't mean you've "screwed up," but rather that the nature of addiction is to take root wherever it can. Watching yourself carefully and being truly honest can help you avoid this pitfall.

Addictions Can Arise Slowly or Quickly

Addiction can grow slow as the grass or hit fast like a punch. There's no one pattern. This is important, because you may think, "I won't develop a problem because I haven't had one before." Crack cocaine may be addictive after just one use. People describe it as one of the best experiences of their lives and they keep chasing that first great high. Alcohol, in contrast, typically takes three to four years to grow from a mild to a serious problem (Schmidt et al. 2000). Addiction may also develop at different points in the lifespan. You may use alcohol just fine until your forties, when your partner dies and you begin abusing alcohol to cope with overwhelming grief. You may go your whole life without an addiction, but as old age sets in you become dependent on medication, a common problem for elderly women. Thus, there's no safety zone from addiction. It can develop or worsen at any time, so the key is to truly listen to what your behavior is telling you.

Addictions May Have Short-Term Positive Benefits

Addiction is clearly not good, but the immediate impact of a substance may feel positive. Alcohol can help you sleep at night. Overeating can feel soothing. Gambling can be exciting. Smoking can help you relax. In fact, one study found that substances gave women a feeling of independence and a sense of purpose otherwise missing in their lives (Taylor 1998). The problem is that these short-term benefits do not last over time. In the long run—the next day or the next week—you feel worse about yourself because you can't stop. People who don't understand addiction may say simple messages such as, "It's just bad for you." It may feel hard to explain that sometimes an addiction does solve some short-term problem. But substances always fail you over time and weaken your life. You can think of it as a classic "bait and switch"—something that seems good is just an illusion.

There Are Various Styles of Addictions

Earlier in this chapter different types of addiction (e.g., alcohol, tobacco) and severity of addiction (abuse and dependence), were described. Getting to know your style of addiction can also be useful. For example, some people binge—they may have "down times," when they're not engaged in the activity, and then go on binges, when they do a huge amount. College students often do this with drinking, waiting until the weekend to *binge* (defined for women as four drinks or more at a time). Other people may be slow and steady, in a more constant addiction. They think about it all the time and find it hard to let a day go by without doing it. Just notice how addiction plays itself out in your life, to help prepare yourself for overcoming it. As they say in war, you must know the enemy to defeat it.

If You Have Relatives With Addiction, You're at Risk

Women are just as likely as men to have genetic vulnerability to addiction (Merikangas 1998). This means that if family members are addicted, there's a strong possibility that you are at risk. Some of the most important research in the past decade has shown that alcoholism, for example, does have a genetic basis (meaning it's passed along in genes to offspring). When you add in the social impact of growing up among people who are addicted—the influence of role models—addiction is even more likely. This does not mean that you can't recover. Regardless of the cause of your addiction (genes, social influence, peers, difficult life history), the process of recovery is the same. Just know that addiction runs in families and that you need to take especially good care to protect yourself if you have this background.

Models of Recovery

If you have an addiction, you may not know where to start. In this section, the goal is to select a next step. No need to think about next month or next year. Just for now, find a way to move forward. Read the options below and put a star next to the one that feels right for you now. You can always change your mind later. The best way to complete this exercise is to involve someone knowledgeable about addiction (e.g., a therapist, sponsor, or doctor). It is a complicated and very important decision, and you should get all the help you can. Also, see the resources at the end of this chapter for more guidance on all three methods.

Please note that this book does not take a position on which way is best. It provides the current options in the addiction field, and suggests ways to decide what might work for you.

Abstinence

Abstinence is the "cold turkey" model, meaning that you give up whatever you're addicted to entirely. It's highly recommended if you have a substance dependence problem. For example, if you're dependent on alcohol, it's wise to stop drinking altogether. This is the tried-and-true method that's been used longest in the addiction field. It's best known as the AA model, but is also the most common model in professional addiction treatment programs—because it works for many people. If you can achieve abstinence, you can learn to rebuild your life without the addiction, finding healthy ways to get your needs met. Note however that for some addictions—such as food, work, or exercise—abstinence may not be possible. You cannot live your life without these activities.

Harm Reduction

Harm reduction means that you commit to engaging in your addiction less, but not to giving it up entirely. It's been called a "warm turkey" model, because it's an alternative to the traditional "cold turkey" abstinence approach (Miller and Page 1991). The goal is to reduce the harm that your addiction is causing. For example, if you use both marijuana and alcohol, you may decide just to give up marijuana for now. Or if you use every day, you may decide to just use every other day. Harm reduction can help you gain control over your addiction, and over time you can cut down more as you feel successful at it. This strategy is often used with people who have co-occurring emotional problems (see chapter 4), who may feel too overwhelmed to commit to abstinence, or who may have been unable to achieve abstinence in the past despite repeated efforts. The idea is that "doing anything is better than doing nothing" (Fletcher 2001, 72).

Controlled Use

Controlled use means that you keep using, but contain it within certain bounds. For example, you have only one drink a day, or gamble only $100 a week. It's also called "moderation management." It avoids an all-or-none position, but establishes when you are within safe limits. It's difficult for many people to stick to these limits, however. Indeed, it's said that every addict already had an experiment with controlled use and failed: many people set "rules" early in their addiction, but can't stick to them and end up even more addicted. However, it's also known that some people with addiction problems are able to succeed at controlled use (Fletcher 2001; McCrady and Langenbucher 1996). It's only recommended for people who have an abuse problem rather than dependence (see earlier in this chapter for definitions). Also, studies show it works best with people who have been addicted for less time (e.g., fewer than ten years), are young (under forty), do not have co-occurring emotional problems (see chapter 4), are employed, have not experienced major losses due to addiction (such as a job or spouse), and, for alcohol, have not had severe withdrawal symptoms when they stopped drinking (McCrady and Langenbucher 1996; NIAAA 2001; Walitzer and Connors 1997).

What is a safe level of use? This has been established only for alcohol, which is the most widely studied addiction. For women, a maximum of one drink per day is considered safe. Just two drinks a day puts women at increased risk of many health problems, such as liver disease (NIAAA 2001). Note that one drink is defined as either five ounces of wine, one shot of hard liquor (measured with a shot glass), or one twelve-ounce beer. For other addictions, you might decide based on talking to a doctor (e.g., for food or exercise addiction) or a therapist (e.g., for shopping or sex). For gambling, you can set a dollar limit that you and your family agree will preserve the family budget. Thus, making a decision about controlled use will depend on the type of addiction, the exact problems you are experiencing, and, typically, getting feedback from others.

Strong Opinions

You should know that people may have very strong opinions about the "right" way to overcome addiction. People who achieved success with abstinence may believe that it's the only approach that really works. People who believe in harm reduction or controlled use may, similarly, have strong feelings about the need for these. Treaters and treatment programs too may have one way of doing things and may tell you it is the only way. You may be interested to know that all three approaches—abstinence, harm reduction, and controlled use—have in fact been found to work for some people (Fletcher 2001; McCrady and Langenbucher 1996). The key is to determine what will work best for you. This will depend on many factors including severity of your addiction, your preferences, your access to support, your family history, and your life problems (e.g., depression).

If you want to read an excellent, highly readable book about the many paths of successful addiction recovery, see Fletcher's *Sober for Good* (2001). She interviewed 222 people who were clean and sober for five or more years, and found that 44 percent credited a traditional 12-step approach (e.g., AA) for their recovery, while 56 percent credited nontraditional methods. Of the 125 people using nontraditional methods, the most common were "multiple paths" (20 percent), "sober on their own" (20 percent), Secular Organization for Sobriety (14 percent), Women for Sobriety (12 percent), and SMART Recovery (10 percent).

Inspiration

In the next section, you'll be encouraged to commit to one of the models of recovery. Before doing so, it may help to remind yourself *why* you are doing it. It's easy enough to make a promise, but keeping one—especially one as challenging as addiction recovery—requires all the motivation you can muster. In one direction is recovery, freedom from addiction, and light; the other direction offers continued addiction, a downward spiral, and darkness.

Describe what inspires your recovery, rating each area on the following scale:

0	1	2	3
Not at all important	A little important	Moderately important	Extremely important

Write a few lines under each area. For example, one woman wrote under "For my children":

My kids—Tanya and Jackson—are my life. I want to give them the best that I can. If I can stop drinking, I can give them the life they deserve. It breaks my heart to think of what my addiction is doing to them.

If you enjoy being creative, you can copy this page and create a small inspiration book from it, adding additional pages with photographs of the people you love or other reminders to help you through recovery. Some people add favorite quotations, poems, songs, or pictures. A photo of yourself can also be a good reminder, such as a picture of you at your best, you as a child, or you at an important life event.

For my children/family   How important? (0 to 3) _____

_____

_____

_____

For my health   How important? (0 to 3) _____

_____

_____

_____

For my spirituality   How important? (0 to 3) _____

_____

_____

For my relationships   How important? (0 to 3) _____

_____

_____

For my work   How important? (0 to 3) _____

_____

_____

To create a better life   How important? (0 to 3) _____

_____

_____

To treat myself with respect   How important? (0 to 3) _____

_____

_____

To give myself the childhood I didn't have   How important? (0 to 3) _____

_____

_____

Other: _____   How important? (0 to 3) _____

_____

_____

_____

_____

A Promise to Yourself

Now it's time to sign off on your commitment—to give your word about the change you want to make. Please fill this out only if you feel truly ready to commit. If you're not ready, that's okay—just being honest is good, and you can seek help from others to decide what you need to do to move forward. You can also decide to return to this once you've finished the rest of this book, rather than completing it now. Be sure to obtain a medical evaluation *before* totally stopping alcohol or drugs. There are serious physical dangers for some people depending on how much and what you've been using.

Remember that when you sign this, you are making a promise to yourself, to your recovery, and to all the people in your life who will be affected by your actions. If you want, take a few moments of silence to connect with what this promise requires of you—how difficult it will be—and also the gifts it will bring you over time. In the exercise below, check off only the *one* choice that you are committing to; leave the rest blank.

I am making a promise to take the following path to heal my addiction:

☐ I commit to **abstinence** from my addiction. This means that I will stop the addiction totally and immediately.

or

☐ I commit to **harm reduction** from my addiction. This means that I will lower my use and later decide whether to reduce it further. (Fill in the amount of reduction you can commit to now; for example, "I will stop my marijuana use totally, and I will drink only one twelve-ounce beer a day.")

_____

_____

_____

_____

or

☐ I commit to **controlled use** of my addiction. This means that I believe I can use safely within limits. Remember: this option is only recommended for people with mild addiction (i.e., abuse rather than dependence). Be sure to re-read the description of controlled use earlier in this chapter to decide whether this is a safe option for you. (Fill in your exact limits, e.g., "I will gamble no more than $100 a week," or "I will have no more than one five-ounce glass of wine a day.")

_____

_____

_____

_____

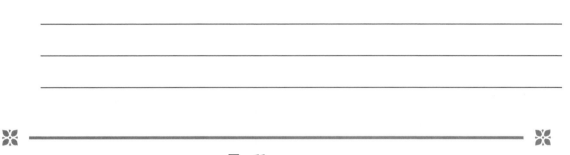

Follow-up

Now that you've made your promise, share it with everyone who can support you in it—your close family and friends, therapist, sponsor, and doctor. The more people you share it with, the more likely you are to achieve success. Each week, fill out the progress log below to see how you're doing. It's important to keep track, as this will give you valuable feedback about whether the plan is working. If you find you cannot keep to your promise, it's strongly suggested that you seek more support—such as AA, therapy, or an addiction program (see the Seek Support section in chapter 6, and the resources at the end of chapters 1 and 2). No matter what happens, don't blame or punish yourself. If you can keep to the promise, that's terrific. If you can't, it simply means that you need more guidance. Seeing your needs clearly and taking care of them is the essence of the recovery process. There's no such thing as "failure" if you can just keep taking the best next step.

For each week, fill in whether you were able to fulfill your promise. Share it with your therapist, sponsor, or other helper.

Yes means you *did it completely.*

No means you *did not do it at all.*

Partially means you were *able to some of it* (describe how much you did).

Were you able to fulfill your promise?			
	Yes	No	Partially (describe)
Week 1 (dates: _____)			

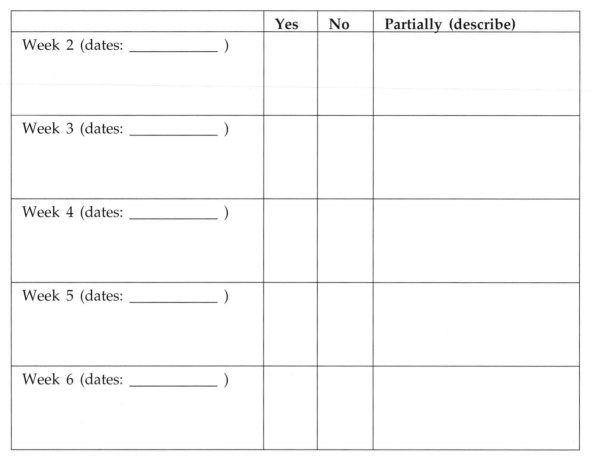

	Yes	No	Partially (describe)
Week 2 (dates: _____)			
Week 3 (dates: _____)			
Week 4 (dates: _____)			
Week 5 (dates: _____)			
Week 6 (dates: _____)			

Continue the log with more dates on a separate piece of paper.

Messages You May Hear

Addictions evoke strong reactions in people. You may hear a variety of messages from people around you. They may be well-meaning, but sometimes you need a way to respond that keeps you anchored to your own truth. At other times, the messages may come from within you, driven by self-hatred, shame, or guilt, and finding a way to respond to these internal messages can help keep you moving forward. Some typical difficult messages follow. After that, you will have a chance to rehearse negative messages you hear and how you might respond.

"You need to just stop using—get over it, already." If stopping were this easy, you would have done it long ago. Recovery requires a lot of support and guidance, and you may not have received enough of that. Learning new coping skills and acquiring more knowledge are keys that can help you stop. Anyone who tells you to "just quit" doesn't understand the nature of addiction.

"Go to AA and you'll be fine. It worked for me." AA and other 12-step programs do work for many people, but for others they do not. Women may have difficulty with some aspects of AA (such as the message, "I am powerless"). If you have serious problems other than addiction—a history of violence or trauma, depression or other emotional issues—AA is likely not going to be enough, because it was never designed to help with these. There are many ways to recover, and AA may or may not be helpful for you. The best advice is to try many different AA meetings, give it your most sincere effort, and then decide. Each woman has her own path.

"You shouldn't take psychiatric medication (or methadone)—that's just another drug of abuse." If you are seeing a reputable doctor who knows your addiction history and prescribes a medication for you, then you are right to take it. People sometimes do not understand that medication, when given appropriately, may help resolve emotional problems that are getting in the way of recovery from addiction. For example, an antidepressant can improve depressed moods. Depression is one of the most common emotional problems in women with addiction, yet is often underrecognized and undertreated (Moras 1998) (see chapter 4). Methadone, similarly, is often misunderstood and unfairly attacked. According to experts and many decades of research, it has been found extremely helpful for some people and can prevent worse addiction problems (Margolis and Zweben 1998). The same holds for other medications that are used to prevent substance abuse, such as naltrexone and Antabuse (Volpicelli et al. 2001).

"Why bother trying? Most addicts return to their addiction." It used to be true that the success rate after addiction treatment was quite low. But the past twenty years have seen the development of much new understanding and many new methods of helping that can save you from a life of addiction misery. Even if you relapse at times, by sticking with the recovery process, you can succeed in the long run. Know that the odds are in your favor, especially if you seek support from people knowledgeable about addiction.

"You need to 'hit bottom' first." This is a common myth, based on the observation that some people do indeed have dramatic recoveries after they suffer major losses (such as a job, partner, or house). However, it's definitely not true that this must happen before recovery begins; many people succeed in recovery without hitting bottom (Fletcher 2001). It's much wiser to get immediate help to prevent problems from worsening. For people with co-occurring emotional problems, such as depression or anxiety, the "bottom" may just keep getting lower until death occurs through suicide, accident, or health problems. For women, these serious risks are much higher than for men (see chapter 1). In short, "raise the bottom"—get help now.

"Unless you're motivated, you won't get better." If you're motivated to work on your addiction, that's terrific. However, you may be interested to know that motivation is often not the starting point for many people who successfully recover. For example, people who are court-ordered to attend addiction treatment do just as well as those who attend voluntarily (NIDA 1999). Some people begin treatment due to external pressure—such as a requirement by their employer or to please a family member—and do just fine once they start. Many people find their motivation increases *after* rather than before they get involved in recovery. Thus, it's best to begin recovery activities even if you don't feel motivated, don't believe in them, or think it's hopeless. As Woody Allen famously said, "Eighty percent of life is just showing up".

Responding to Difficult Messages

Try rehearsing how you would respond to a message about addiction that you find difficult. Below, write out the message, and then how you would respond to it *within your own mind*. You do not have to say it out loud to anyone. Just practice being supportive of yourself, getting clear in your own mind what you really believe.

Message: "_____ ."

Your response: _____

_____

_____

_____

_____

_____

_____

☎ Resources

The resources below provide further guidance on the three models of recovery described in this chapter, and on self-help groups of all kinds. Most are free. See also the resources on addiction in chapter 1.

Models Of Recovery

Abstinence

Women for Sobriety Adaptation of the 12 steps for women	215-536-8026	www.womenforsobriety.org
Alcoholics Anonymous	800-637-6237	www.alcoholics-anonymous.org
Cocaine Anonymous	310-559-5833	www.ca.org
Narcotics Anonymous	818-773-9999	www.na.org
Marijuana Anonymous	800-766-6779	www.marijuana-anonymous.org
16 Steps for Discovery and Empowerment Holistic approach to addiction	406-273-6080	www.charlottekasl.com
Smart Recovery Non-spiritually based self-help	440-951-5357	www.smartrecovery.org
Secular Organizations for Sobriety/Save Our Selves	323-666-4295	www.secularsobriety.org
LifeRing Secular Recovery	510-763-0779	www.unhooked.com

Harm Reduction

Harm Reduction Coalition	510-444-6969	www.harmreduction.org

Controlled Drinking/Moderation Management

Moderation Management Network	212-871-0974	www.moderation.org
DrinkWise	888-816-2736	www.med.ecu.edu/pharm/ drinkwise/wise.htm

Self-Help for Other Addictions

Gamblers Anonymous	213-386-8789	www.gamblersanonymous.org

Workaholics Anonymous	510-273-9253	http://people.ne.mediaone.net/wa2/
Overeaters Anonymous	505-891-2664	www.overeateranonymous.org
Nicotine Anonymous	415-750-0328	www.nicotine-anonymous.org
Co-Dependents Anonymous	602-277-7991	www.codependents.org
Debtors Anonymous	781-453-2743	www.solvency.org
Sexaholics Anonymous	615-331-6230	www.sa.org
Sexual Compulsives Anonymous	800-977-HEAL	www.sca-recovery.org
Sex and Love Addicts Anonymous	781-255-8825	www.slaafws.org

CHAPTER 3

Exploring Your Life Patterns

As you heal from addiction, you will see that recovery is not just about giving up something, such as alcohol, compulsive shopping, or overeating. Far more, it is a process of discovering who you are. Addiction arises out of unmet needs—and thus much of the work ahead is to identify and fulfill your needs. It's about giving voice to wishes and feelings you may have hidden away for a long time. It's about taking good care of yourself, finding your truth, and becoming aware. Changing a habit may take as little as a month (Covey 1990), but this deeper journey to your real self will be lifelong.

Addiction is always an escape, and as such it detaches you from yourself. You lose your groundedness and sense of confidence. Addiction is an illusion: a seemingly good thing in the beginning that somehow in the end goes bad. You lose yourself to your addiction, and after a while it owns you. You may literally live and die for it. The focus of an addiction is, moreover, almost always something physical: a drink, a drug, money, possessions, or physical pursuits such as excessive sex or exercise. By trying to grasp too much onto these material things, you lose your grip on other, nonmaterial sides of life that may be even more fulfilling—such as love of nature, sense of purpose, healthy relationships, and creativity. But you're not sick, lazy, crazy, or bad—addiction is never about some irredeemable flaw in you as a person. Rather, it's a sign that you've gone off track, chased the wrong dream.

In this chapter, the goal will be to explore life issues that may be related to your addiction. Five typical themes for women are:

- ✖ Body and sexuality

- ✖ Stress

- ✖ Thrill-seeking

- ✖ Relationships

- ✖ Trauma and violence

For each theme, some ideas will be discussed, a brief personal story will be provided, and then you will be asked to explore the theme in your own life. Resources are provided if you want to find out more. Some topics will likely ring more true for you than others, and indeed, that's the purpose of this chapter—to help you look beyond the addiction to unmet needs you may have. In the next chapter, emotional problems will be described—such as depression, anxiety, and eating disorders.

Keep in mind that exploring these life problems does not mean they are the "real" issue behind your addiction, or that they caused your addiction. In earlier times, a mistake in the treatment field was to search for an underlying cause rather than helping people work on the addiction itself; the idea was that if you resolved your psychological conflicts, the addiction would disappear on its own. This is known to be false (Margolis and Zweben 1998). Addiction is a disease that needs direct attention and care, regardless of what other problems you have.

Yet it is also true that women often have life issues that are associated with addiction. By addressing these, as well as the addiction itself, you are more likely to get better. The idea is to help you with all parts of your life, not just the addiction. Women often suppress their own needs to focus on others, and may lose touch with themselves. In chapters 6 through 9, ways of healing will be discussed, but for now the goal is just to get to know your life patterns more fully. As with the rest of this book, feel free to skip around in this chapter to what interests you.

Life Strengths

Before starting on your life difficulties, it may be helpful to identify your strong sides—the qualities that come naturally to you, your talents and gifts. These might include, for example, sense of humor, persistence, or the ability to face your feelings. It's just as important to notice what's going right as to notice what's wrong. And don't be modest—there's no need to hide your strengths. Really own them and delight in them. The work on life difficulties may be painful, so it's good to first connect with your strengths. Everyone, addicted or not, has a mix of strengths and difficulties. *Try this exercise even if you think you don't need it, or it feels stupid, or you think you can't.* Give it your best shot!

Rate each strength below using the following scale. Really notice what's good about you.

0	1	2	3
Not at all	A little	Moderately	Extremely

Connecting with others. I have a gift for making connections with people. I find friends easily, and enjoy being with people. _____

Creativity. I'm good at art, dance, music, writing or some other creative pursuit. I like to play with imagination and possibility. _____

Political action. I try to make a difference in the larger world. I may help with advocacy (such as promoting the rights of women, lesbians, or children). I may volunteer in my community at a library or soup kitchen, for example. _____

Attractiveness. I am physically beautiful or charming. People are drawn to me because they find me appealing. _____

Sense of humor. I can find fun in almost any situation. I like to laugh and notice the quirks and absurdities in life. _____

Survival skills. I survived painful life experiences, such as a dysfunctional family or child abuse. Or I may have completed schooling or done a job that was difficult. I am a survivor. _____

Persistence. I can follow through on commitments even when I don't feel like it. I have a sense of will and make an effort to improve things. _____

Self-care. I take care of myself—eating right, exercising, getting annual check-ups, and taking care of my physical environment, such as my home. _____

Physical ability. I'm good at sports or other physical activity (without being addicted to it). _____

Social support. I have one or more people in my life who love me and genuinely want me to get better. I believe they'll help me when I ask, and be there emotionally when I need them. _____

Helping others. I'm good at caring for others, such as children, pets, elderly, or others who need my help. _____

Self-esteem. I have some positive feelings about myself. This may include pride in my achievements, valuing my personal qualities (e.g., honesty, integrity, warmth), or believing that I'm a good person. _____

Spirituality. I am a deeply spiritual person. I sense larger forces and can tap into that positive energy. I may or may not be religious, but I have this gift of awareness. _____

Intelligence. I "get it"—whether it's formal learning (mental intelligence), knowing how to relate to people (social intelligence), or dealing with feelings (emotional intelligence). I may have one of these strongly, or all of these somewhat. _____

Ability to face my feelings. I can face feelings that are painful and deal with them. I may manage my feelings in a variety of ways: crying, thinking about them, or just letting myself experience them. _____

Ability to communicate. I can say what I think and feel without hurting myself or others. This is sometimes called "assertiveness"—expressing myself without being either passive (getting "walked on") or aggressive (attacking people). _____

Financial resources. I have money available that can help me obtain therapy and other resources for overcoming addiction. _____

Others:

_____

_____

_____

_____

_____

Can't find any? Some people feel they have no strengths. They may hate themselves too much to notice anything positive, or they may never have learned to see what's good in them. But, everyone has strengths—no exceptions! Try taking this exercise to someone who knows you, such as a friend, partner, sponsor, or therapist. Often they can see good qualities that you may not.

Life Difficulties

Now it's time to explore—and honor—your areas of difficulty. If you can, go through each theme and complete the exercises. Remember not to blame yourself. The goal is to understand yourself with an open heart and mind.

In fact, did you know that both strengths and difficulties can feed addiction, and both can heal addiction? You may think that strengths are great and difficulties are bad. In fact, there is a deeper truth: both can be good, bad, or a mix. For example, perhaps one of your strengths is connecting with others. This may promote recovery by allowing you to seek support from others. But it may also hinder recovery: you may drink or drug more when you are around people; you may ignore an addiction problem if people around you don't notice it; or you may value others' needs above your own and thus delay efforts to help yourself.

The same holds for difficulties. For example, perhaps you use alcohol to manage stress. This can certainly be negative—it perpetuates your addiction. But it can also promote your recovery if you use stress to truly respond to your needs. You may see that stress is a message that must be heard rather than drowned with alcohol. Perhaps the stress is telling you that your job is too high-pressure, that you need more balance in your life, or that you have taken on other people's problems too much. By using stress as a clue to your inner life, you gain insight.

In short, as you explore your life difficulties, try not to judge yourself as "good" or "bad." You are a complex human being, and can use any difficulty to promote healing from addiction or to perpetuate it. You have the power to choose growth rather than destruction. However, it's not okay to keep abusing substances. If you found in chapter 2 that you have an addiction, *the addiction itself is not positive.* The goal throughout is to overcome the addiction.

Theme 1: *Body and Sexuality*

A woman's relationship to her body is complex, and may have strong connections to addiction. A woman's worth is often defined by her physical appearance, and she may become overly concerned with her body as a way to win attention, power, or love. Addiction may serve these purposes (Kasl 1990). The use of substances to increase sexual response is common, for example. One study found that sexual dysfunction was the single best predictor of women's alcohol problems over a five-year period (Covington and Surrey 1997b). Ironically, however, alcohol actually decreases sexual functioning in women (Blume 1997). Addiction may also be a way to force the body into an impossible ideal—through overexercising, purging, or excessive plastic surgery. Weight loss is one of the most common reasons for women's smoking and their abuse of diet pills (Bulik and Sullivan 1998). Normal body changes such as development during adolescence, menopause, or aging may feel upsetting, and addiction may become a way to cope. Many women in addiction treatment report a connection between their menstrual cycle and substance abuse; and indeed, women with serious premenstrual problems have higher rates of addiction than those without (Blume 1997b). Addiction itself often leads to the neglect of normal body needs, such as regular medical exams and a healthy diet. The use of substances to cope with medical illness (such as alcohol to numb physical pain) is also well known (Heinemann 1997). Women who sell their bodies through prostitution often use substances as a way to detach from the degradation they feel. Eating disorders are also quite common among women with substance abuse issues (Bulik and Sullivan 1998). Addiction to sex may be a way to feel loved; as Kasl notes, a woman may decide, "If I can't get love, I'll take sex" (1992, 101). Finally, a history of childhood physical and or sexual abuse is very common among women with addiction. Such mistreatment of a girl's body can lead to enduring problems, including body self-neglect and addictive self-mutilation (e.g., cutting, burning).

A Personal Story

Jennifer got a lot of attention for her appearance while growing up. She was blond and cute, and people were drawn to her. During her teen years she became overly concerned with her body image. She began using diet pills and smoking as a way to stay thin, and at times would purge and use laxatives. She developed a view of herself as someone people only liked because of her looks. She enjoyed the attention yet felt disappointed that her appearance was the main thing people noticed. With men she also had mixed feelings: liking their interest, but uncomfortable with the sexuality involved. She would drink to reduce her discomfort with sex. By her mid-twenties her use of smoking, alcohol, and diet pills began to concern her.

How About You?

Now it's time to take a look at your own life.

Step I: Exploration

How do you feel about your body? Draw an X on the line below to indicate your view:

Hate	Neutral	Love
my body	about my body	my body

How do you feel about your sexuality? Draw an X on the line below to indicate your view:

Hate	Neutral	Love
my sexuality	about my sexuality	my sexuality

Step II: Making the Connection

Now see whether there is a link between your body and sexuality issues and your addiction. **Is your addiction a way to:**

☐ Feel more sexual (e.g., using alcohol or cocaine to lower your inhibitions)?

☐ Lose weight (e.g., by smoking, abusing diet pills, or overexercising)?

☐ Feel attractive (e.g., through compulsive shopping)?

☐ Mold your body into an ideal image (e.g., by overexercising or excessive plastic surgery)?

☐ Numb out physical feelings (e.g., taking opiates to reduce pain)?

☐ Punish your body (e.g., cutting or other self-mutilation)?

☐ Cope with body changes, such as your menstrual cycle, illness, or aging?

☐ Feel loved (e.g., compulsive sex to feel connected to others)?

☐ Other:_____

☐ Other:_____

In your own words, how do body and sexuality issues relate to your addiction?

_____

_____

_____

_____

_____

_____

�֎ ——————————————————————————————————— ✖

Self-Awareness Summary

Overall, how much are your body and sexuality issues related to addiction:

In the present?

0	1	2	3
Not at all	A little	Moderately	Extremely

In the past?

0	1	2	3
Not at all	A little	Moderately	Extremely

✖ ——————————————————————————————————— ✖

Theme 2: *Stress*

Stress means feeling pressure or tension—from money problems, conflicts with people, or a noisy environment, for example. It's the number one cause of relapse in substance abuse, even after long periods of abstinence (NIDA 2001). Moreover, women more than men report that their addictive use of a substance began after a stressful event (Blume 1997a). Low amounts of stress can actually improve performance: think of how a deadline at school or work may spur you to work better. But high stress can lead to substance use as a way to relax, such as the businesswoman who overworks and then "needs" several drinks to wind down. Stress also leads to physical illness: the more stress, the more likely you are to become ill. Ongoing or extreme stress results in permanent biological changes that make you more reactive to future stress, more easily "triggered" in everyday life. Stress leads to emotional problems as well, such as depression and anxiety. In fact, many of the emotional problems that you'll read about in chapter 4 are known to become worse with stress. Women tend to have especially high stress around balancing work and family, taking care of others, and being less powerful than men in the workplace (Blum and Roman 1997). The most common stress women report is lack of time (McKenna 1998).

With extremely stressful events, such as a rape, serious car accident, or fire, a person may develop posttraumatic stress disorder (PTSD) (see chapter 4 to explore whether you have this). PTSD is an emotional disorder that usually requires professional help, and is known to be common among women with addiction (Najavits 2002).

Many aspects of your life can lead to stress, however, even if they seem small: not getting enough sleep, boredom, lack of privacy, conflicts with neighbors, a difficult boss. Indeed, even *positive* events are stressful if they require you to adapt to a new identity: graduation from school, a new baby, a promotion at work (Miller, Smith, and Rothstein 1993).

One of the key ideas in managing stress is learning your own patterns. It's been said that some people are "horses" while others are "butterflies"—some can tolerate a lot of stress while others can't (Miller, Smith, and Rothstein 1993). In AA, the acronym "HALT" is used to identify common stressors that lead to using: **H**ungry, **A**ngry, **L**onely, **T**ired. It's important to become exquisitely aware of your stress level—like the gauge on a car that goes into the red zone when overheating. At that point you need to protect yourself by finding ways to calm down without substances. For each person, these ways differ. The goal is to discover what works for you: deep breathing? socializing? taking a walk? watching TV? (See the growth exercise Soothing Yourself in chapter 9 for suggestions.)

A Personal Story

Adrienne took care of everyone around her. She was a single parent to her three children, all under age twelve. She helped take care of her mother, who was sick with cancer, and she worked part-time as a teacher's aide for a seventh-grade class. At times she felt she was losing her mind. She had no time to herself, and the demands on her seemed never to end, morning to night. She felt guilty if she complained, but inside she was a ticking time bomb. Little things would set her off: she would blow up at a store clerk who was too slow, or sometimes at her kids, which she felt terrible about. There seemed to be no way out. She needed the money from her job and couldn't change careers. There was no one to help her. She found herself drinking more and more. What started out as a drink when she got home became half a bottle of wine, and then a pint of hard liquor. Often during the day she would crave her "drinking break." She kept promising herself that she would cut down.

How About You?

Now it's time to take a look at your own life.

Step I: Exploration

What are the current stresses in your life (in the past twelve months)?

Negative Stressors

☐ Money (e.g., debt, poverty, or loss of income)

☐ Job (e.g., too many demands or hours, conflicts with people, or a job change)

☐ Caretaking of others (e.g., children or parents)

☐ Lack of time

☐ Boredom

☐ Death of someone close to you

☐ Not enough sleep

☐ Bad neighborhood (e.g., a lot of drugs or crime)

☐ Lack of privacy (e.g., your own space)

☐ Too many things to do

☐ Physical illness

☐ Loss of partner (e.g., through divorce or separation)

☐ Discrimination (e.g., for being minority, female, or lesbian)

☐ Noise

☐ Too much travel (e.g., a difficult commute or frequent work trips)

☐ Legal problems (e.g., arrest or jail)

☐ Major relationship problems (e.g., sexual problems, fights, or domestic violence)

☐ Other:_____

☐ Other:_____

Positive Stressors

☐ A new baby

☐ Major relationship change (e.g., marriage, engagement, or new partner)

☐ Preschool children

☐ A new job or school

☐ Moving

☐ Promotion (e.g., school graduation or a new job role)

☐ Vacation, major trip, or holiday season

☐ Other:_____

☐ Other:_____

In general, how stressful is your life these days?

0	1	2	3
Not at all stressful	A little stressful	Moderately stressful	Extremely stressful

Step II: Making the Connection

Now see whether there is a link between your stress and your addiction. **Is your addiction a way to:**

☐ Tune out the stress?

☐ Relax?

☐ Cope (e.g., get through the day)?

☐ Forget about a specific problem (e.g., finances or health problems)?

☐ Make it seem like everything's okay?

☐ Compensate (e.g., thinking "I need to use after all these problems")?

☐ Celebrate (e.g., when you finish a project)?

☐ Hide your stress from others?

☐ Help you get the job done (e.g., drinking so you can write)?

☐ Other: _____

☐ Other: _____

In your own words, how does stress relate to your addiction?

_____

_____

_____

_____

_____

_____

Self-Awareness Summary

Overall, how much is your addiction related to stress:

In the present?

0	1	2	3
Not at all	A little	Moderately	Extremely

In the past?

0	1	2	3
Not at all	A little	Moderately	Extremely

See the resources at the end of this chapter if you want to pursue the topic of Stress further.

Theme 3: *Thrill-Seeking*

For some people, addiction begins in thrill-seeking—wanting to party, escape boredom, feel "cool." While more common in males than females, thrill-seeking is found especially among younger people in their teens and twenties. It is believed to be genetically based, meaning that you're likely born with it as part of your personality. People who seek thrills typically have a variety of high-risk behaviors, including heavy drinking, problem gambling, unsafe sex, speeding while driving, multiple sexual partners, drug use, extreme sports (e.g., bungee-jumping), and criminal behavior (e.g., Powell et al. 1999). Certain drugs, such as the party drug ecstasy (MDMA), are used more among people with this trait (Miles et al. 2001). For some people, it's just a phase, while for others it can lead to a serious addiction. For women, thrill-seeking increases the risk of sexual assault (Combs Lane 2001). Thrill-seeking may be part of wanting to fit into a certain crowd or of overcoming the boredom of a dull job or town. Thrill-seeking is not necessarily a life difficulty; the search for pleasure is understandable. But, when it is extremely strong or leads you to take dangerous risks in which you do not adequately protect yourself, then it's a problem.

A Personal Story

Jana goes to rave parties where almost everyone gets blitzed on ecstasy and alcohol. There are lots of different pills, and half the time she doesn't know what she's taking. Her motto is, "I'll try anything once." She and her friends begin partying around midnight and come home at dawn. She's twenty-three years old and feels this is the time of her life. She and her friends dress cool, act cool, live cool. But at a recent rave she was raped by a guy she didn't know. It freaked her out and made her wonder whether she was too involved in a scene she couldn't control.

How About You?

Now it's time to look at your own life.

Step I: Exploration

How much of a thrill-seeker are you?

0	1	2	3
Not at all thrill-seeking	A little thrill-seeking	Moderately thrill-seeking	Extremely thrill-seeking

How dangerous is your thrill-seeking behavior (i.e., how risky is it? how likely is it to result in physical harm)?

0	1	2	3
Not at all dangerous	A little dangerous	Moderately dangerous	Extremely dangerous

Step II: Making the Connection

Now see whether there is a link between your thrill-seeking and your addiction. **Is your addiction a way to:**

☐ Feel "cool"?

☐ Escape boredom?

☐ Connect with fun people?

☐ Party?

☐ Get thrills?

☐ Feel young?

☐ Make sex more intense?

☐ Make conversations more intense?

☐ Feel more alive?

☐ Have some danger in your life?

☐ Rebel?

☐ Get a kick from doing something illegal?

☐ Live for the moment?

☐ Lower your inhibitions (e.g., for kinky sex)?

☐ Imitate someone you admire (e.g., a rock star, a celebrity, or an older sister)?

☐ Other: _____

☐ Other: _____

In your own words, how does thrill-seeking relate to your addiction?

_____

_____

_____

_____

_____

_____

_____

❈ ═══ ❈

Self-Awareness Summary

Overall, how much is your thrill-seeking related to addiction:

In the present?

0	1	2	3
Not at all	A little	Moderately	Extremely

In the past?

0	1	2	3
Not at all	A little	Moderately	Extremely

❈ ═══ ❈

Theme 4: *Relationships*

Relationships may be the single greatest influence on women's addiction. Addictions are often started and maintained in relationships. Indeed, many women report that their initiation into substance use occurred with a partner or substance-abusing family (Boyd and Guthrie 1996). There are many ways that relationships and addiction may be linked for women, including using to soothe loneliness, fit in, or please a partner sexually. Addiction to relationships themselves may also be a major problem—staying with someone you know is bad for you or being unable to be alone (Covington 1988).

One popular theory holds that women's primary motivation in life is relationships (much more so than for men). Thus it's no surprise that addiction and relationships so often go together for women. Indeed, the substance itself often becomes the most important relationship once someone is heavily addicted: "Alcohol was my true love, I never went to bed without Jack Daniel's"; "My most passionate affair was with cocaine"; "Food was my mother, my friend, whom I turned to for solace and comfort, who was always there for me when I needed it" (Covington and Surrey 1997, 338). Throughout the life span, substances may replace relationships that are damaged or weak. Higher rates of substance abuse have been found, for example, among young women who are estranged from their families, middle-aged women who are divorced or having serious conflicts with their partners, and older women who are widowed (Gomberg 1997).

Your partner may be one of the biggest influences on how much you use and whether you relapse (Connors, Maisto, and Zywiak 1998). This "partner factor" is consistently found to be more important for women than for men. Men are more likely to relapse alone, for example, while women are more likely to relapse in the presence of a partner (Rubin, Stout, and Longabaugh 1996). It's also been observed that women with addiction have difficulty connecting with other women (Lichtenstein 1997), which reduces their level of support and may intensify the overimportance of a partner. Finally, addiction itself typically worsens relationships, as it may lead to neglecting your children while high, having fights, or isolating.

A Personal Story

Judy is in a passionate but difficult relationship. She and her boyfriend have stormy fights and sometimes don't speak for days. He is jealous and won't allow her to have men friends or leave without telling him where she's going. She loves him, but can't stand the constant surveillance. They keep breaking up, then getting back together. They do a lot of cocaine together. She feels as addicted to the relationship as to the cocaine—the intense highs make it seem worthwhile until the next fight. She feels she can't live with him and can't live without him.

How About You?

Now it's time to look at your own life.

Step I: Exploration

Answer the questions below using the following scale. Think of the totality of your relationships: friends, family, sponsor, therapist, boss, colleagues, etc.

0	1	2	3
Not at all	A little	Moderately	Extremely

How much do your relationships feel *supportive*? (i.e., people are caring and warm, listen to you, give good advice, want you to succeed) _____

How much do your relationships feel *destructive*? (i.e., people undermine you, abuse you, use you, or make you feel bad about yourself) _____

How much do your relationships feel *neutral*? (i.e., you are very isolated with few or no relationships, or your relationships don't really make much difference) _____

How much of the time do you *feel bad* about your relationships (e.g., guilt, shame, anger, anxiety, or conflict) _____

How much of the time do you *feel good* about your relationships (e.g., joy, fun, or closeness) _____

Step II: Making the Connection

Now see whether there is a link between your relationship issues and your addiction. **Is your addiction a way to:**

- ☐ Feel closer to a partner who uses?
- ☐ Fit into your family or community?
- ☐ Grieve a loss, such as divorce, death, or a child leaving home?
- ☐ Please a partner sexually?
- ☐ Feel relaxed around people?
- ☐ Feel more sociable (e.g., witty, fun)?
- ☐ Soothe loneliness?
- ☐ Feel energy or love because these are missing from your relationships?
- ☐ Belong (e.g., drinking when everyone else is)?
- ☐ Tolerate violence from a partner?
- ☐ Cope with rejection?
- ☐ Change yourself when you feel "too big" in a relationship (e.g., angry, sexual, powerful, or needy)?

☐ Change yourself when you feel "too small" in a relationship (e.g., fearful, childlike, dependent, or vulnerable)?

☐ Avoid being alone (e.g., addiction to a relationship)?

☐ Other: _____

☐ Other: _____

In your own words, how do your relationship issues relate to your addiction?

_____

_____

_____

_____

_____

_____

_____

_____

Self-Awareness Summary

Overall, how much are your relationship issues related to addiction:

In the present?

0	1	2	3
Not at all	A little	Moderately	Extremely

In the past?

0	1	2	3
Not at all	A little	Moderately	Extremely

See the resources at the end of this chapter if you want to pursue the topic of relationships further.

Theme 5: *Trauma and Violence*

Did you know that *most* women in addiction treatment (55 percent to 99 percent) have suffered trauma? *Trauma* means an experience of physical harm, such as rape, fire, or life-threatening illness. Even seeing someone else physically hurt is a trauma, for example, finding a dead body or watching a shooting. Fifty-one percent of American women suffer a trauma during their lifetime, typically child abuse, natural disaster, or seeing others hurt (Kessler et al. 1995). Women also may be perpetrators of violence against others, and this too can take a toll on emotional well-being, making them feel guilty or afraid of their own actions (Hien and Hien 1998). Indeed, many women in prison for violent assault against others have a history of addiction.

Many women are not helped to cope with these overwhelming events and may try to just forget about them. But the memories may keep coming back in nightmares or images they can't escape. They may feel angry, depressed, and worthless. Addiction numbs the pain, whether drinking, drugs, or any other compulsive activity such as overeating or overexercising (Zweben, Clark, and Smith 1994). Indeed, for most women, the trauma or violence occurs first and addiction develops later (Miller, Downs, and Testa 1993). Yet when women enter treatment, they often are not asked about this history; no one helps them connect these horrible events with their addiction (Brown, Stout, and Gannon Rowley 1998). The good news is that if they are given help for both addiction and trauma, they tend to get better (Najavits 2002).

A Personal Story

Linda has many addictions: cocaine, alcohol, self-cutting, and food. She grew up in a violent home where the children were beaten. She says, "We had all this chaos happening in my family. Drugs were a great way of numbing. Drugs stopped the pain. You wanted to escape, and it felt like there was no other way to escape. You just needed something to get away from it all. It was a way of protecting myself, like a shield. Drugs gave me the courage, the strength, to deal with things most people never have to deal with."

How About You?

Now it's time to look at your own life.

Step I: Exploration

Identify your history of trauma through the questions below. Use "maybe" if you're not sure (e.g., you were too young to remember but suspect it happened). **Important:** *If it's upsetting to fill this out, stop immediately. Do not continue until you seek* *support from a therapist or other helper. Remember a key message of this book is to take care of yourself!*

In your lifetime, have you suffered any of the following experiences, or seen them happen to someone else?

Child physical abuse (e.g., hitting that caused bruises or injury)	Yes	No	Maybe
Child sexual abuse (e.g., being molested, touched, or forced into any sexual activity)	Yes	No	Maybe
Child neglect (e.g, not enough to eat, inadequate shelter)	Yes	No	Maybe
Domestic violence (a partner who hurt you physically)	Yes	No	Maybe
Crime victimization (e.g., rape, holdup)	Yes	No	Maybe
Serious accident (e.g., car crash, chemical spill, or fire)	Yes	No	Maybe
Life-threatening illness (e.g., cancer)	Yes	No	Maybe
Natural disaster (e.g., hurricane, earthquake)	Yes	No	Maybe
War	Yes	No	Maybe
Captivity or kidnap	Yes	No	Maybe
The threat *of any of the events above,* even if it wasn't completed (e.g., threat of being raped or murdered)	Yes	No	Maybe
Violence by you (e.g., you physically hurt someone, such as abusing a child, murdering someone, or attacking someone with a weapon)	Yes	No	Maybe
Other upsetting events: _____ _____ _____ _____ _____	Yes	No	Maybe

If you're not sure whether an event was trauma or violence, ask your therapist about it, or call the resources at the end of this chapter for help.

Step II: Making the Connection

Now see whether there is a link between your trauma or violence and your addiction. **Is your addiction a way to:**

☐ Shut off feelings or memories of the event?

☐ Feel more (e.g., you're numb or detached)?

☐ Punish yourself (e.g., believing it was your fault)?

☐ Get through it (e.g., drinking to tolerate domestic violence?)

☐ Soothe yourself?

☐ Feel powerful (e.g., the event made you feel powerless)?

☐ Get back at someone (e.g., rebelling against a parent who hurt you)?

☐ Commit "slow suicide" (e.g., you don't care if you live or die)?

☐ Other: _____

☐ Other: _____

In your own words, how does your trauma or violence relate to your addiction?

_____

_____

_____

_____

_____

_____

Self-Awareness Summary

Overall, how much is your trauma or violence related to addiction:

In the present?

0	1	2	3
Not at all	A little	Moderately	Extremely

In the past?

0	1	2	3
Not at all	A little	Moderately	Extremely

See the resources at the end of this chapter if you want to explore the topic of trauma and violence further.

Self-Understanding

What did you find out? Hopefully, this chapter helped you explore whether your addiction connects to unmet needs—the need to respect your body, manage stress better, find thrills in safe ways, develop more supportive relationships, or cope with trauma or violence.

If your Self-Awareness Summary for any of the five life issues had ratings *in the present* of 1 or more, you may benefit from learning how to cope better—without the use of substances. Learning new coping skills can occur through chapters 6 through 9 in this book, reading other books on healthy coping, seeking professional help, and/or contacting the resources listed in this chapter. If you had any ratings *in the present* of 2 or 3 it is strongly suggested that you seek professional help. You're suffering a great deal and may not have the skills yet to resolve the issue on your own.

The Self-Awareness Summary ratings *in the past* were designed to help you explore the history of your addiction—whether it arose in the context of unmet needs in the past.

The more aware you are of these life issues and the more you work to resolve them, the more likely you are to overcome your addiction. As always, however, you need to reduce or eliminate your substance abuse at the same time. Resolving these unmet needs cannot be a reason to justify continued addiction.

The next chapter encourages you to explore emotional problems that are common in women with addiction. Then, the rest of the book offers growth exercises to help you cope with the issues you identified. It is said that knowledge is power—and perhaps the most important knowledge of all is who you really are inside.

☎ Resources

Body and Sexuality

National Eating Disorder Association	800-931-2237	www.nationaleatingdisorders.org
Weight-Control Information Network	877-946-4627	www.niddk.nih.gov/health/nutrit/win.htm
Food and Drug Administration, Office of Women's Health	301-827-0350	www.fda.gov/womens/default.htm
Food and Drug Administration Consumer Hotline	800-532-4440	www.fda.gov
American Society for Reproductive Medicine	205-978-5000	www.asrm.org
North American Menopause Society	440-442-7550	www.menopause.org
Administration on Aging—National Aging Information Center	202-619-7501	www.aoa.dhhs.gov
National Institute on Aging Information Center	800-222-2225	www.nih.gov/nia
Older Women's League	800-TAKE-OWL	www.owl-national.org

For sexual addiction, see the resources in chapter 1. Also, there are a very large number of associations to help with illnesses such as cancer, asthma, diabetes, AIDS, (for example, the American Cancer Society). For a list, search the Internet or ask your librarian.

Stress

American Institute of Stress	914-963-1200	www.stress.org
Office of Alternative Medicine Clearinghouse	888-644-6226	www.nccam.nih.gov
For information on treatments often used for stress—e.g., meditation, acupuncture, herbs		

For traumatic stress, see the end of this chapter.

Stress Related to Care-Giving

National Maternal and Child Health Clearinghouse	888-275-4772	[no website]
Children of Aging Parents	215-945-6900	[no website]
Family Voices For people taking care of children with special needs	888-835-5669	www.familyvoices.org
Eldercare Locator	800-677-1116	www.eldercare.gov

Relationships

Join Together To help communities fight addiction	617-437-1500	www.jointogether.org/jto/
Al-Anon and Alateen For family members of people with addiction	800-356-9996 (Al-Anon) 800-344-2666 (Alateen)	www.al-anon-alateen.org

For sex/love addiction see the resources for body and sexuality earlier in this chapter.

Trauma and Violence

International Society for Traumatic Stress Studies Referrals for trauma treatment, and education	847-480-9028	www.istss.org
Sidran Foundation Trauma information, support	410-825-8888	www.sidran.org
Cavalcade Videos Videos on trauma for patients and therapists	800-345-5530	www.pacificsites.com/~cavideo
National Victim Center Infolink Information on crime victimization	800-FYI-CALL	www.ncvc.org/infolink/main.htm
National Centers for PTSD Extensive literature on trauma, education, and assessment	802-296-5132	www.ncptsd.org

National Clearinghouse for the Defense of Battered Women	215-351-0010	[no website]
National Domestic Violence Hotline	800-799-SAFE	www.ndvh.org
National Resource Center on Domestic Violence	800-537-2238	www.pcadv.org
Many Voices A trauma survivors newsletter	513-751-8020	www.manyvoicespress.com
The Healing Woman A trauma survivors newsletter	408-246-1788	www.members.aol.com/healingw.htm

CHAPTER 4

Dual Recovery

This chapter explores *co-occurring disorders*: the idea that many addicted people also have an emotional problem such as depression, eating disorder, or anxiety disorder. *Co-occurring* means "happening at the same time" as the addiction. It's also called *dual diagnosis* or *double trouble*, for two disorders.

Most substance abusers have a co-occurring disorder; and this pattern is more common in women than in men (Blume 1997b; Kessler et al. 1997; Regier et al. 1990).

Why is this an important idea? Because if you get help for your emotional problem, you're more likely to succeed in addiction recovery. This is called *dual recovery*—working on both the addiction and the emotional problem at the same time. It is now widely recommended. The old way (still heard in some treatment programs) is, "Get clean first, and then we'll deal with your emotional problem." The new view is that working on both at the same time, from early in treatment, is likely to be more helpful (CSAT, in press; Weiss, Najavits, and Mirin 1998).

If you are depressed, for example, you may need therapy or medication to relieve the depression—which in turn can help you control your addiction. Indeed, the emotional problem usually arises first, the addiction second—a pattern suggesting *self-medication* (using a substance to cope with emotions) (Kessler et al. 1996).

Once an emotional disorder is identified you may say, "Now I get it!" Something clicks, and you see yourself and your recovery needs more clearly. Yet many people go their whole lives with an emotional problem that is never named. They may genuinely want to work on their addiction, but repeatedly fail to get clean and sober. When the emotional problem flares up, they're back into the addictive cycle: using to feel better, then feeling worse, using more, and so on. They may wonder why others can recover but they can't. Does this sound familiar?

Sadly, people with co-occurring disorders also have more life problems than people with addiction alone—more homelessness, hospitalization, criminal behavior, and suicide, for example (Knowlton 1995). What can never be fully measured is their sheer suffering—the low self-esteem, the disruption of a normal life, the years of pain.

Most people never get help for emotional problems, even though it could make a world of difference. Fewer than half are in treatment (Kessler et al. 1996). If you suspect you have an emotional problem, it is *strongly* suggested that you seek help. These disorders are illnesses, just like diabetes or asthma. Some people don't believe in them because they can't see them. But they are real, and they can be helped.

You may have hidden your emotional problem, even from family and friends. Many people do not understand emotional problems. They may say, "How weird," "Get over it already," or "That's an excuse—your problem is addiction." When people talk this way, they're not aware that an emotional problem needs medical attention. They don't understand that if you could just snap out of it, you surely would! No matter how much they love you, they may get frustrated and not know what to do. It's also true that your emotional problem may be causing hardship to the people around you. Your children may be especially affected, even though they can't put it into words. If you have unresolved emotional problems, your children are more likely to develop them too.

In the following pages, some major disorders will be described, with a focus on those most common in women. You can see whether any apply to you. You may have no disorder, one, or more than one. Many women have several. But don't feel you have to decide for yourself. The idea is to get a first impression and then, if you want, ask a professional for feedback. If you suspect, *even slightly*, that you have a problem, it's wise to have someone evaluate you. It's always better to be wrong or to catch a problem early than to wait until it's full-blown.

Some people fear the word *disorder*. They think it means "crazy" and "forever." They may have grown up in a culture where emotional problems were not discussed. In older times, an emotional problem was viewed as a black mark against the family, a sign of serious mental illness. People would often blame the person who had it. However, it's now clear that emotional disorders are common. In fact, 50 percent of people in the U.S. have an emotional disorder during their lifetime (Kessler et al. 1994). Many people who have them appear normal but are suffering inside. The past twenty-five years have seen great progress in understanding how common emotional problems are and how to treat them. You can find out, get help, and move on; you don't have to stay stuck in quiet isolation.

Some Encouragement

How does it feel to explore co-occurring disorders? Some find it a relief. One woman, learning that she had posttraumatic stress disorder, said:

> "At first I thought, 'Oh no, not another condition,' but then I was relieved to find I had something with a name. I thought it was just me—I'm crazy. But I can deal with this now. It's different when you don't know, but when you find out, it's like a person with cancer—you can work on it. Now I can put down the cocaine and work on what's behind it."

Other women feel upset, seeing that they now have more to work on than they thought. They may find that it takes a while to adjust to this new understanding.

There is much hope in recognizing your emotional problems. It means you can move forward. One of the worst parts of addiction is feeling as though it's all your fault, that you've "screwed up." With co-occurring disorders, you get the sense that it's more complicated. Sure, it would have been better not to get addicted. And yes, it's true that you need to take serious action now to work on the addiction. But perhaps you needed more than addiction treatment or AA alone. Maybe you needed help with your emotional problems too. Many women never got that.

Most of all, you should know that it's never too late, no matter what your age or circumstances. You can choose a first step that is comfortable for you: getting a screening to see if you have the disorder, reading about it, searching on the Internet for information, finding a support group of others with the same problem, or obtaining therapy or medication. You have options. You have the rest of your life in front of you.

Try to take as positive an attitude as you can toward yourself. Give yourself the gift of compassion for your experience. Only you know what you have struggled with and how hard it all was. It takes courage to explore these issues. Whatever comes up, you can find a way to take good care of yourself now.

As always, if you become upset while reading this chapter, stop. You can go to the next chapter and come back to this when you feel ready. Don't push through, believing that you "should be able to handle this." Listen to where you are and respect that.

Identifying Emotional Problems

As you read through the nine emotional problems described here, **check any boxes that fit you *in the present*.** If any are unclear, put a question mark beside them. If you want, write a "P" next to those you had in the past.

If an emotional problem clearly doesn't apply to you, skip to the next one. Also, certain facts such as rates and subtypes, are given for each disorder. You don't have to read this material unless you find it helpful. Some people like a lot of information, while others prefer just the basics.

If you have children, you may want to go back over this chapter a second time to see whether your children have any of these problems. If you think they might, it's strongly advised that you get help for them now, before they get worse.

When answering the questions, try to think of a time when you were not using substances. This may be difficult if you have been using for a long time, but you should know that addiction itself can create emotional problems, such as feeling depressed or anxious, or seeing things that aren't there. Similarly, some medical conditions and even medications can create these problems. Here too, an evaluation by a professional can help sort it out. You may want to show that person how you answered the questions in this chapter.

All of the emotional problems in this chapter are derived from the *Diagnostic and Statistical Manual of Mental Disorders, 4th ed.* (APA 1994), and they represent standard definitions in the field. The language, detail, and organization have been simplified a great deal for readability. Note that the term *addiction* in this chapter refers to substance addiction, as that has been studied most with co-occurring disorders.

Depression

Depression means that you feel sad, blue, down. While everyone feels this way at times, people with depression can't shake it. They feel depressed most days. For some, depression can be so severe that they feel life is not worth living, they are worthless, and there's no hope. They may become so depressed that they can't get out of bed. The signs of depression are:

☐ You feel sad, hopeless, or empty most of the time.

☐ You have less interest and pleasure in things than you used to.

☐ You eat too much or too little.

☐ You sleep too much or too little.

☐ You're either so "speeded up" or "slowed down" that others notice it.

☐ You are tired, lacking energy.

☐ You feel worthless or guilty.

☐ You have difficulty thinking or making decisions.

☐ You think a lot about death; you may want to kill yourself.

If you have many of these problems for two weeks or more, it's called *major depression*. Major depression may occur once or several times during your life. If you have a few of these problems lasting a long time (two years or more), it is low-level depression, or *dysthymia* (meaning "negative mood"). Women are known to be at risk for *double depression*, suffering both major depression and dysthymia. Other depressions common in women are *seasonal depression*, which occurs only at one time of year (typically winter, due to less light being available during the day), and *postpartum depression* (depression that occurs after having a baby). Sometimes depression occurs after other major life events as well, such as divorce or losing a job.

In some cultures, depression may be expressed by other terms, such as "nerves" in Latino cultures, "imbalance" in Asian cultures, or "heartbreak" in American Indian cultures (APA 1994, 324). In children, depression may appear as pretending to be sick, not wanting to go to school, clinging, worrying that a parent may die, getting into trouble at school, or being grouchy and negative (NIMH 2000). These signs may be difficult to see as depression—they can look like bad behavior or "just a phase," but here, too, getting a professional evaluation is important.

How About You?

How much do you think you currently suffer from depression?

0	1	2	3	?
No depression	Mild depression	Moderate depression	Extreme depression	*Can't rate (not sure/don't know)*

If you answered 1 or more on this scale, you may be interested to read more about depression in the next section. If you answered 0 ("no depression"), go to the next disorder.

More About Depression

Depression is one of the most common emotional problems in women, with over 20 percent of women (one in five) experiencing it in their lifetime (Kessler et al. 1994). (As they say, if you're sitting in a group of five, one of you likely has it!) Moreover, women have double the rate of depression as men. The combination of depression and addiction is also more common in women than in men (Schuckit 1998). Almost one-third of depressed people have substance addiction, highlighting how often the two go together (Regier, et al. 1990). In women with alcohol dependence, 49 percent have major depression and 21 percent have dysthymia (Kessler et al. 1997).

Sadly, two-thirds of depressed people never seek treatment, even though treatment works 80 percent of the time (NIMH 2000). Experts say, "Depressive Illness is among the most common and destructive of illnesses prevalent in the United States today.... Most do not know they have a treatable illness. Most blame themselves and are blamed by others" (NFDI 2001). Depression can also impact the people around you. It's been said that for every depressed person, three to four people around them are directly affected.

If you do seek treatment, it's important to obtain help from a clinician who understands mental health. Often, people are given the wrong medication (e.g., sleeping pills rather than antidepressants), too low a dose of medication, or a potentially addictive medication. There is still much to be done to improve treatment services for depressed people.

Why is depression so common in women? The answer is a combination of physical and social factors. Physical factors include biochemical imbalance in the brain, hormones, thyroid problems, menstrual problems, pregnancy, menopause, miscarriage, and a family history of depression. Social factors include the typical issues women face, such as balancing work and home, single parenthood, taking care of children and aging parents, poverty, and discrimination. Women who were sexually or physically abused as children or are victims of domestic violence also have high rates of depression.

Bipolar Disorder/Mania

Bipolar disorder means "extreme moods." You're on an emotional roller coaster, from feeling very low to feeling very high. The low extreme is depression (described in the section above), the high extreme is called *mania*. Mania means that you are speeded up way beyond your normal self. Mania does not come from any substance, but rather from your brain chemistry going off-kilter. Mania and depression may come and go suddenly or slowly, or they may both happen at the same time. Some people just have mania (without any depression). The signs of mania are:

☐ You feel unusually "high," energetic, or elated, without any substance.

☐ You are extremely irritable.

☐ You need much less sleep.

☐ You have racing thoughts or speech.

☐ You are much more active than usual (e.g., a frenzy of work).

☐ You have exaggerated beliefs about how great you are (e.g., "I can run the United Nations").

☐ You get distracted very easily.

☐ You get into trouble (e.g., spending all your money in a shopping spree).

☐ You have poor social judgment (e.g., giving advice to passing strangers).

If you have several of these for at least one week (without being high on any substance) it is *mania*. Or, if you are hospitalized for these behaviors, even if they don't last a full week, that too would be mania. If you have these problems to a lesser degree, it is *hypomania*. Both mania and hypomania refer to a pattern of behavior that is different from your normal self; indeed, so different that people who know you notice it. You may even dress differently and engage in unusual behaviors (e.g., traveling suddenly to a distant city). There are many different combinations of depression and mania; you can obtain information on your own pattern if you seek a professional evaluation. Often, a manic state is triggered by a stressful event, such as losing your job.

If you are in a state of mania, you may not recognize that you are ill and may refuse treatment. Later, after the mania is over, you may have great regrets about your behavior. You may have hurt family members without knowing it, through excessive spending, reckless driving, or impulsive romantic relationships.

How About You?

How much do you think you currently suffer from mania?

0	1	2	3	?
No mania	Mild mania	Moderate mania	Extreme mania	*Can't rate (not sure/don't know)*

If you answered 1 or more on this scale, you may be interested to read more about mania in the next section. If you answered 0 ("no mania"), go to the next disorder.

More About Bipolar Disorder/Mania

Bipolar disorder is less common than depression. But it's one of the most common disorders to co-occur with substance addiction. Indeed, most people with bipolar disorder (56 percent) have substance addiction (Regier et al. 1990). If you have bipolar disorder, you're six times more likely to have addiction than someone without bipolar disorder. Women have lower rates of bipolar disorder than men, but both women and men are equally likely to have the combination of bipolar disorder and addiction. Among women with alcohol dependence, 7 percent have mania; among men it's 6 percent (Kessler et al. 1997).

People with the combination of bipolar disorder and substance addiction are more likely to attempt suicide, to need hospitalization, and to have less success in treatment than people with bipolar disorder alone (Weiss, Najavits, and Greenfield 1999). However, if the person is willing to take medication for the bipolar disorder, it can make a huge difference. Medication is one of the best treatments for bipolar disorder, although psychotherapy also can be helpful.

Posttraumatic Stress Disorder

Posttraumatic stress disorder (PTSD) may develop after you experience a horrible event involving physical harm—such as rape, fire, domestic violence, or terrorist attack. Such events are called *traumas*, and PTSD means, literally, "after-trauma-anxiety-problem." (See the section Trauma and Violence in chapter 3 for more about traumas.) If you have PTSD, you're overwhelmed by intense feelings and memories of the horrible event that you lived through. It may seem as though the disaster is happening over and over in your mind, and you can't shut it off. About one-third of people who experience a trauma develop PTSD (Kessler et al. 1995). The signs of PTSD are:

☐ You suffered a trauma (see the section Trauma and Violence in chapter 3).

☐ You felt overwhelmed when the trauma happened (intense fear or horror).

☐ *Intrusion.* Memory of the trauma keeps coming into your mind even though you don't want it to (nightmares; "*flashbacks*" that feel like the trauma is happening again; or being *triggered*—you feel an intense reaction when reminded of the trauma).

☐ *Avoidance and numbing. Avoidance* means you push the trauma out of mind (e.g., you don't want to think about it, you avoid reminders, or you have trouble remembering some of what happened). *Numbing* means you feel much less than you used to (e.g., you feel detached, you have less interest in activities, or you have no sense of a future).

☐ *Arousal*: Your mind and body are on high alert (difficulty sleeping and concentrating, scanning the room for danger, anger outbursts, and intense startle reaction).

If you checked off all five boxes, and the problem has lasted more than a month, it's *PTSD*. If you have the problems for less than a month, it's *acute stress disorder*.

With PTSD, you may also have other painful feelings: blaming yourself; guilt for surviving (e.g., if others died); intense shame; impulses to hurt your body; despair and loss of trust; or feeling damaged. Some people have a delayed reaction, meaning they only develop problems six months after the trauma or later. PTSD develops most often after a violent assault (Breslau et al. 1998).

In children, PTSD may appear as repeated "danger" play. For example, a child in a car accident may keep showing crashes with toy cars. Also, children may have physical complaints rather than emotional upset.

In some people (although it's quite rare), severe trauma may lead to *dissociative identity disorder*, in which you have different personalities and switch between them, often feeling out of control in this switching. This used to be called *multiple personality disorder*, as in the popular movie *The Three Faces of Eve*.

How About You?

How much do you think you currently suffer from PTSD?

0	1	2	3	?
No PTSD	Mild PTSD	Moderate PTSD	Extreme PTSD	*Can't rate (not sure/don't know)*

If you answered 1 or more on this scale, you may be interested to read more about PTSD in the next section. If you answered 0 ("no PTSD"), go to the next disorder.

More About PTSD

Women have double the rate of PTSD as men, and many women in addiction treatment have current PTSD (33 percent to 59 percent) (Kessler et al. 1995; Najavits, Weiss, and Shaw 1997). Unfortunately, they are rarely evaluated for it or given treatment even though effective treatments exist (Brown, Stout, and Gannon Rowley 1998). The most common trauma for women in addiction treatment is childhood physical or sexual abuse. They often have PTSD for many years. It's as if one tragedy is piled on top of another: suffering a horrible event, feeling terrible, and using substances to cope. Indeed, most women who have both develop PTSD first and addiction later. "Numbing the pain" is a common phrase (Najavits, et al. 1998).

If you have both PTSD and addiction, you need to protect yourself from further harm. For example, you may keep getting into abusive relationships, or you may not take good care of your body. You may find it hard to trust people and want to leave treatment early when you're upset. Learning skills to gain control over your feelings is one of the key steps in treatment, and eventually, when you are ready, perhaps telling the story of what happened to you (Ruzek, Polusny, and Abueg 1998). You may be encouraged to know that you can recover from PTSD if you get professional help from someone trained to work on it. For some, treatment may be short (e.g., if you had a single trauma as an adult); for others, it may take longer (e.g., if you had many traumas as a child). Either way, you *can* get over it.

Eating Disorders

If you have an eating disorder, it means you use food to express emotional pain. There are different eating problems: eating too much (*binging*), eating too little (*restricting*), getting rid of food after you've eaten it (e.g., throwing up), or a combination of these. You can't see yourself clearly, and you believe your body is too fat. Like in a fun-house mirror, you see yourself in a distorted way. What you can't see is that the problem is not your body—it's about all sorts of emotional issues, such as trying to feel in control, trying to get people to like you, and trying to feel good about yourself. You can never feel good through what you eat or don't eat, so you remain in an endless cycle of frustration and pain.

There are two basic types of eating disorders. The first, *anorexia*, means that you are intensely afraid of gaining weight. The signs of anorexia are:

☐ You refuse to keep your body at a normal weight.

☐ You have an intense fear of getting fat, even though you're underweight.

☐ You have an extremely distorted view of your body, believing you're fat no matter what people tell you and obsessing constantly about your weight.

☐ You miss three of your menstrual periods in a row.

Note that some anorexics just restrict their food. Others restrict, but also at times binge on lots of food and then purge to get rid of it (e.g., by throwing up or using laxatives).

The second type of eating disorder is *bulimia*. If you have this, you are in a constant cycle of bingeing on too much food, then trying to get rid of it. The typical signs of bulimia are:

☐ You binge repeatedly (you eat a much larger amount of food than is normal, and you feel that you can't stop).

☐ After bingeing, you make up for it by getting rid of the food (e.g., you throw up, use laxatives, fast, or overexercise).

☐ You go through this cycle often (at least twice a week for three months).

☐ You obsess about your body and your weight.

If you binge but don't try to get rid of the food after eating, it's called *binge eating disorder*.

You may be in denial about your eating disorder. Sometimes it's only family or friends who see the problem and try to get you help. Most eating disorders (90 percent) occur in women, and most occur in developed countries where people have enough to eat but where issues of control, success, and appearance are prominent. If you have an eating disorder, you're at high risk for all sorts of medical problems, and about 10 percent of anorexics die from the illness.

How About You?

How much do you think you currently suffer from an eating disorder?

0	1	2	3	?
No eating disorder	Mild eating disorder	Moderate eating disorder	Extreme eating disorder	*Can't rate (not sure/don't know)*

If you answered 1 or more on this scale, you may be interested to read more about eating disorders in the next section. If you answered 0 ("no eating disorder") go to the next disorder.

More About Eating Disorders

Bulimics are more likely to have substance addiction than anorexics. Indeed, about one-third of bulimics report addiction, particularly to alcohol and stimulants. The use of substances often begins as a way to lose weight. It also may serve to reduce inhibitions about eating, and to cope with guilt and other negative feelings about having eaten too much (Bulik and Sullivan 1998).

Women are more likely to have an eating disorder than men. Among women in treatment with an eating disorder, 3 percent to 50 percent have a substance addiction (Bulik and Sullivan 1998).

Generalized Anxiety Disorder

If you have *generalized anxiety disorder* (GAD), you worry most of the time. You may worry about your job, finances, children, health, household chores, car repairs, being late, or just about anything else. The worry takes over your day and is upsetting, but you can't stop. It's more than just the minor worrying that everyone has at times. You may seek constant reassurance from people, but it doesn't really make a difference. You may have felt this way all your life, and even if it gets better at times it feels like it's part of who you are. Here too, as with all the other emotional problems, treatment is available. GAD does not have to be "who you are." The signs of GAD are:

☐ You worry most of the time, and this has continued for at least six months.

☐ You can't control your worrying.

☐ Most days, you have three or more of the following (for children, just one is needed):

    ☐ You feel keyed up, restless.

    ☐ You get tired easily.

    ☐ Your mind goes blank, or you can't concentrate.

    ☐ You're irritable.

    ☐ You have a lot of tension in your muscles.

    ☐ You have sleep problems.

Note that worry occurs in many emotional disorders. If you have an eating disorder, for example, you are single-mindedly focused on the fear of gaining weight. In

GAD, however, you worry about all sorts of things and the worry itself is the problem.

There may be cultural differences in GAD. In some cultures, people express anxiety mainly through their bodies, having a lot of physical complaints. In other cultures, anxiety may be more mental, such as obsessing about everyday life. Also, children may show the disorder in different ways. They may redo tasks to get them "just right"; they may be too focused on their performance at school or sports even when they're not being evaluated; they may worry about catastrophes such as earthquakes or nuclear war. They may seek a lot of approval from adults, and may be overly "good," not acting like just regular kids.

How About You?

How much do you think you currently suffer from GAD?

0	1	2	3	?
No GAD	Mild GAD	Moderate GAD	Extreme GAD	*Can't rate (not sure/don't know)*

If you answered 1 or more on this scale, you may be interested to read more about GAD in the next section. If you answered 0 ("no GAD"), go to the next disorder.

More About Generalized Anxiety Disorder

GAD is two to three times more common in women than in men. The combination of GAD and addiction is about equal in both sexes, however. Among women with alcohol dependence 16 percent have GAD (Kessler et al. 1997). Most women with GAD and addiction do not receive treatment for their anxiety, however (Moras 1998).

Obsessive-Compulsive Disorder

If you have *obsessive-compulsive disorder* (OCD), it means you feel tortured by upsetting thoughts that you can't stop (*obsessions*), or by the need to keep doing an action that you can't stop (*compulsions*). Examples of obsessions include the thought that you are "dirty" after shaking people's hands, the image of hurting your child, the idea that you have to have things in perfect order, or the thought that you left the stove on. These are not just passing thoughts, but occur over and over and are extremely upsetting. Examples of compulsions include the need to keep washing your hands, checking things, repeating words to yourself, counting, or praying. It's as if you have a rule book that no one else has. You feel that you absolutely have to do the action so that you can feel less upset. You do the activity far beyond what anyone else would do. You don't do it because you enjoy it, but because you're terribly afraid that if you don't, something awful will happen. Often, people have both obsessions and compulsions, and these are connected. For example, you're obsessed with the thought that your hands are dirty, so you feel compelled to wash them until your skin is raw. Many people are superstitious at times, as in the childhood rhyme about walking on the sidewalk ("step on a crack, break your mother's back"). But in OCD the superstitions take over your life. The signs of OCD are:

☐ You have either obsessions, compulsions, or both.

Obsessions:

    ☐ You have upsetting thoughts that keep coming into your mind.

    ☐ Your obsessive thoughts are not based in reality (e.g., there's no reason to believe you left the stove on).

    ☐ You try to get rid of the thoughts.

    ☐ You know that the thoughts are your own (no one is forcing you to think them).

Compulsions:

    ☐ You feel you have to keep repeating something (e.g., handwashing or counting).

    ☐ You're trying to prevent some awful event from happening.

☐ You are aware that the obsession or compulsion doesn't make sense.

☐ You are very upset by the obsession or compulsion, it takes up a lot of time (more than one hour a day), or it interferes with your life.

Note that in many emotional disorders people may obsess or feel compelled to keep doing something. For example, in substance addiction it is common to obsess about your drug of choice and feel compelled to keep using. In OCD, however, you are obsessing about something that doesn't make any sense and doesn't bring you any pleasure.

At some point, most adults with OCD realize that the obsession or compulsion is out of hand. However, it may take a while to see this. Often children are not aware they have a problem. Unless their parents see it and get them help, they may suffer for many years, trying to hide their OCD.

OCD can lead you to avoid many normal life activities in an attempt to prevent the obsession or compulsion from happening. Your life may become very narrow.

Some people have an emotional problem called *obsessive-compulsive personality disorder*. This is different from OCD; for more on this disorder, see the section Personality Disorders later in this chapter.

How About You?

How much do you think you currently suffer from OCD?

0	1	2	3	?
No OCD	Mild OCD	Moderate OCD	Extreme OCD	*Can't rate (not sure/don't know)*

If you answered 1 or more on this scale, you may be interested to read more about OCD in the next section. If you answered 0 ("no OCD"), go to the next disorder.

More About Obsessive-Compulsive Disorder

OCD is equally common in women and men. Among people with OCD, 33 percent have a substance addiction (Regier et al. 1990). The substances of choice are usually ones to help calm down—alcohol, sedatives, antianxiety pills. You may also seek a lot of reassurance from people as a way to feel better. For women, OCD typically occurs during their twenties, while for men, it occurs when they're younger. When under stress, your OCD may get worse.

Phobias

If you have a phobia, you're extremely afraid of something. It might be just about anything: blood, snakes, heights, bridges, public speaking, choking, or dating, for example. Many people are afraid of such things at one time or another, but for you, it's an extremely intense fear that has clearly made your life worse. For example, public speaking is known to be the most common fear that people have. But for you, it's so intense that you turn down promotions at work just so you won't have to do it. You might be so afraid of flying that you drive for two days straight to avoid getting on a plane. It's not that you want to live like this, but your fear is so extreme that you can't live a normal life. You will do just about anything to avoid facing your fear. It feels unbearable. The signs of phobia are:

☐ You have an intense fear of something, way beyond what most people would have. Check off your fear(s):

   ☐ Certain animals or insects (e.g., snakes or bugs)

   ☐ Nature (e.g., storms, heights, or water)

   ☐ Blood or injury (e.g., you faint when you see blood or an open wound)

   ☐ Daily life situations (e.g., bridges, tunnels, elevators, flying, driving, enclosed spaces, or public transportation)

   ☐ Social situations (e.g., having conversations, eating in public, using public restrooms, dating, or public speaking)

   ☐ Other (e.g., choking, vomiting or becoming ill):

   _____

   _____

☐ You're always very anxious when you have to face the thing you fear.

☐ You know your fear is way out of bounds, but you can't control it.

☐ You go out of your way to avoid having to face your fear.

☐ Your fear is very upsetting, or has a major impact on your life (e.g., you have no friends because you are so afraid of talking to people).

Note that you only have a phobia if you actually have to face the particular situation. For example, you may be extremely afraid of snakes, but unless the fear impacts your life in some clear way, you don't have a phobia. You may live in a city and never see snakes, so your life is not severely impacted by snakes. Similarly, if your job doesn't require you to do public speaking, you wouldn't have a public speaking phobia (even if you're deathly afraid of it) because it has no impact on your life.

There are also cultural differences around fears. In some cultures, magic or spirits are feared. This wouldn't be a phobia unless you're much more upset about it or severely impacted than other people from your culture. Children are only seen as having a phobia if it lasts more than six months. (Children have many fears, but these usually only last a few months.) *Agoraphobia* is a fear of places that you can't get away from, because you're afraid of having a panic attack in those places. This is covered in the next section, Panic Disorder.

How About You?

How much do you think you currently suffer from phobia?

0	1	2	3	?
No phobia	Mild phobia	Moderate phobia	Extreme phobia	*Can't rate (not sure/don't know)*

If you answered 1 or more on this scale, you may be interested to read more about phobias in the next section. If you answered 0 ("not at all phobic") go to the next disorder.

More About Phobias

Phobias are much more common in women than in men. For women, the most frequent phobia is fear of animals; among men it's fear of heights (Curtis et al. 1998). More important than the type of fear is the number of fears you have: the more you have, the worse your life is.

Among people with phobia 23 percent have a substance addiction (Regier et al. 1990). Women, however, have higher rates of this dual diagnosis than men do. Among people with alcohol dependence, for example, 31 percent of women have a phobia, compared to 19 percent of men (Kessler et al. 1997).

Panic Disorder

If you have panic disorder, it means you suddenly get intense attacks of anxiety. They're terrifying, and you may feel like you're going crazy, losing control, having a heart attack, or dying. The panic attacks seem to come out of nowhere, and you don't understand why they're happening. You want to escape. You may think you have a physical illness, even though doctors tell you that you don't. You may blame yourself, believing that you're weak. The signs of panic disorder are:

☐ You have panic attacks. A *panic attack* means:

  ☐ You suddenly feel extremely anxious.

  ☐ You have four or more of the following, all within ten minutes:

    ☐ Heart pounding, or speeded-up heart rate (palpitations)

    ☐ Sweating

    ☐ Shaking or trembling

    ☐ Shortness of breath, feeling smothered

    ☐ A choking feeling

    ☐ Chest pain or discomfort

    ☐ Nausea or upset stomach

    ☐ Feeling dizzy, light-headed, or faint

    ☐ Feeling unreal or detached from yourself

    ☐ Fear of losing control or going crazy

    ☐ Fear of dying

    ☐ Numbness or tingling

    ☐ Chills or hot flashes

☐ Some of your panic attacks seem to come out of nowhere ("out of the blue").

☐ After at least one of your panic attacks, you were very worried about having another or about what it meant (e.g., you thought, "I'm crazy"), or you changed your behavior because of it for at least one month.

Many people with panic attacks also have *agoraphobia*, which means that you avoid any situation that you fear may bring on a panic attack. For example, you may avoid crowds, public transportation, going outside, bridges, or elevators. You dread having a panic attack and being unable to escape, or having no one there to help you. Eventually, you may find your life becomes very narrow as you avoid normal activities, such as shopping, work, and travel. If you are forced to be in one of your feared situations, you feel extremely upset. You may find it easier to endure these situations if you have a companion. The word *agoraphobia* is from an old Greek word meaning fear (*phobia*) of the marketplace (*agora*); i.e., fear of crowds.

You may also have *limited symptom attacks*, in which you have fewer than four of the panic attack signs listed above. Another pattern includes *situational panic attacks*:

when you first have panic disorder, the attacks come out of nowhere, but eventually certain situations may also bring them on (e.g., when you're driving a car). Finally, you may develop general anxiety, even when you're not having an actual panic attack. For example, you may worry a lot about your health or about losing someone close to you.

Note that some people have panic attacks as part of other emotional problems, including phobias and posttraumatic stress disorder. If you have a phobia, for example, you may have panic attacks when you're faced with the thing you fear, such as snakes or blood.

How About You?

How much do you think you currently suffer from panic disorder?

0	1	2	3	?
No panic disorder	Mild panic disorder	Moderate panic disorder	Extreme panic disorder	*Can't rate (not sure/don't know)*

If you answered 1 or more on this scale, you may be interested to read more about panic disorder in the next section. If you answered 0 ("no panic disorder"), go to the next disorder.

More About Panic Disorder

Women are two to three times more likely than men to have panic disorder. Among people with panic disorder, 36 percent also have substance addiction. Among women with alcohol dependence, 12 percent have panic disorder and 19 percent have agoraphobia (Kessler et al. 1997). Panic disorder has been found to run in families, and is believed to be at least partly genetically based.

Personality Disorders

A *personality disorder* means you have a long-standing pattern of behavior that is causing serious problems in your life. There are a variety of personality disorders. For example, you may be extremely sensitive to criticism from other people and thus avoid getting into any relationships. Or you may repeatedly get into trouble with the law. Or you may feel very dependent on other people, not making decisions for yourself and not standing up for yourself. They are called "personality disorders" because they are ongoing personal styles that stay the same over time. Some emotional problems covered earlier in this chapter may come and go (e.g., major depression, panic disorder, or PTSD). Personality disorders, in contrast, are always there—until you get help for them. All personality disorders begin when you are either a teen or a young adult.

It's important to know that your personality has many sides. Some are terrific—you may be kind to people, a hard worker, or artistic, for example. Everyone has good qualities. Having a personality disorder doesn't mean you're a bad person or that your whole personality is negative. It just means that in addition to your positive sides, there is a side that is causing serious problems in your life. It may feel like people don't understand you, or that you don't know why things keep turning out wrong.

Finally, it's important to note that what may be a problem in one culture may not be in another. For example, if you grew up in an Asian or Hispanic community where family relationships are extremely close, it may be perfectly acceptable—in fact desirable—that you're highly dependent on your family. It may be expected that you will make decisions by first talking to your family, and that you will live with your family even as an adult. The same behavior in someone who grew up in a typical Caucasian home in the U.S., where independence is valued, might be a problem. Thus, when deciding whether or not you have a personality disorder, you should take into account how people in your community act. It's only when it is very different from most people around you and when it's causing serious problems in your life that it's a problem.

The general signs of personality disorder are listed below, followed by brief descriptions of several common personality disorders. It may feel hard to decide if you have one (more so than for other disorders in this chapter). Asking the opinion of a trusted family member, friend, or therapist can help.

Note: **Check off the boxes below only after you've read the description of each personality disorder.** Otherwise, it will be difficult to fill out accurately.

- ☐ You have a long-standing pattern of behavior that differs from that of most people in your community. This shows up in two or more areas:

    - ☐ Thinking (how you view yourself, people, and life)

    - ☐ Feelings (their intensity and range)

    - ☐ Relationships

    - ☐ Impulse control (i.e., dangerous behavior)

- ☐ Your pattern of behavior occurs across many situations; it feels stuck or rigid.

- ☐ Your pattern of behavior causes you a lot of upset, or leads to serious problems (e.g., in work or relationships).

- ☐ You have had the pattern of behavior since your teen or early adult years, and it has been the same over time.

Types of Personality Disorders

You may have one or more of the personality disorders described here. When reading each description, try to get an overall feel for it, you don't have to have each of the signs. Try to think of whether the overall description feels like it fits you and whether it causes you problems. Also, think about how others would describe you.

☐ *Avoidant Personality Disorder.* You're afraid of people. You don't feel good enough, and believe that you will be criticized or rejected. You may try to be invisible in social situations, and expect that no matter what you say, people will disapprove. You actually very much want to have relationships, but you need a lot of reassurance that you will be liked. You feel inferior, unappealing, and socially inept. You may avoid many social situations, including dating, job interviews, and group activities.

☐ *Dependent Personality Disorder.* You have trouble making decisions without a lot of advice and reassurance. You may want others to make decisions for you, such as where to go to school. You feel uncomfortable disagreeing with people because you fear they won't like you. You need to be in a relationship at all times, and are extremely worried about being left to take care of yourself. You may volunteer to do things that are unpleasant (such as always being the one to clean up) because you want others' approval. You doubt your abilities and find it hard to start projects on your own.

☐ *Obsessive-Compulsive Personality Disorder.* You are very focused on order, perfection, and control. You are so consumed with details, rules, lists, and schedules that you lose sight of the big picture. You try so hard to be perfect that you may have major difficulty completing tasks. You're so devoted to work that you leave little time for leisure and friendship. You are extremely scrupulous about ethics and morality. You're a pack rat, finding it hard to throw things out. You have difficulty delegating work to others unless they submit exactly to your way of doing things. You have difficulty spending money and tend to be an oversaver. People might say you're stubborn.

☐ *Borderline Personality Disorder.* Your life feels unstable—in relationships, moods, and how you see yourself. You engage in damaging impulsive behavior (e.g., reckless driving, spending, sex, binge eating, or substance abuse). You feel empty a lot of the time. You have intense feelings that change quickly, such as anger and sadness. Your relationships are unstable: you may love someone for a while and then hate the person. You have difficulty seeing yourself the same way over time and may suddenly switch jobs or friends. You have repeated impulses to harm your body, such as cutting, burning, or suicide threats.

☐ *Antisocial Personality Disorder.* You repeatedly do things that could get you in trouble with the law, such as getting into physical fights, destroying property, using a weapon, hurting animals, assaulting people, theft, robbery, reckless driving, or conning people. You rarely plan ahead, and may have frequent debts and job changes. You may view people negatively, believing they're just out for themselves. You've had many of these behaviors since you were younger than fifteen years old.

☐ *Schizoid Personality Disorder.* You are a loner. You don't enjoy relationships of any kind, including family or sexual ones. You have little interest in activities and your emotional style is detached. You don't have strong emotions such as anger or joy. Other people's opinions of you don't matter much. If you have relationships they're likely to be with your immediate family only.

☐ *Paranoid Personality Disorder*. You are highly suspicious of people, even when there is little evidence of actual danger. (Note: If you've been seriously hurt through child abuse, domestic violence, or other real events, this disorder does not apply to you.) You continually question whether people are loyal. You don't confide in people because you believe they'll hurt you. You bear grudges and find it hard to forgive. You suspect your partner is unfaithful without any real reason. You're quick to interpret people's comments as put-downs or attacks, even when they didn't mean them that way.

How About You?

How much do you think you currently suffer from one or more personality disorders?

0	1	2	3	?
No personality disorder	Mild personality disorder	Moderate personality disorder	Extreme personality disorder	*Can't rate (not sure/don't know)*

If you answered 1 or more on this scale, you may be interested to read more about personality disorders in the next section. If you answered 0 ("no personality disorder") go to the next section.

More About Personality Disorders

Personality disorders are extremely common among people with substance addiction (35 percent to 91 percent) (Brooner et al. 1997; Weiss et al. 1998). Of the different types, antisocial personality disorder is most associated with addiction. Indeed, it's the single most common co-occurring disorder—84 percent of people with antisocial personality have an addiction (Regier et al. 1990). Many more men than women have it, but rates for women are still high. Among women dependent on alcohol, for example, 29 percent have antisocial personality or related disorders (Kessler et al. 1997).

Borderline personality disorder is the next most common among women with addiction. Among women in substance abuse treatment 10 percent have borderline personality disorder (Brooner et al. 1997). Many other personality disorders have not yet been studied much.

Other Emotional Problems

Several other emotional problems are not included in this chapter. Some are much less common in women (e.g., narcissistic personality disorder), others are relatively rare in general (e.g., fire-setting), and others are so extremely disabling that you'd likely already know if you had them (e.g., schizophrenia). Some problems are not covered because they're not as central to addiction recovery (e.g., sleep disorders, or sexual and gender identity problems). Others are seen primarily in medical settings (somatoform disorders and factitious disorders). If you believe you have an emotional problem that is not described here, be sure to ask a mental health professional to help you identify what it might be.

Keys to Dual Recovery

Did any emotional problems in this chapter feel like they fit? If so, you may want to pursue *dual recovery*. Dual recovery means working on *both* the substance abuse and the emotional disorder at the same time. It's currently a widely recommended approach (Ries, in press). It can make your addiction recovery more likely to succeed.

Dual recovery might mean getting a medication or therapy to relieve your depression, eating disorder, or phobia, for example, while also doing AA or other addiction work. It may involve exploring how your addiction and emotional disorder are linked: how they arose over time, why they go together, and how your substance use may have been an attempt to cope. If you're in a treatment program where you're getting help for only one problem (just the addiction or just the emotional disorder), you owe it to yourself to seek out the resources at the end of this chapter. You don't have to end your current treatment, but you can add to it so that you get help for both. You deserve the best possible care.

Some key concepts in dual recovery are as follows.

If you feel in danger of hurting yourself or others, get help now. Many of the emotional problems in this chapter are highly associated with suicide (e.g., depression, bipolar disorder, posttraumatic stress disorder, and borderline personality disorder). You may also have impulses to hurt others. These are signs that you're in a great deal of pain and need immediate help. No matter how awful life seems when you're in this dark place, it doesn't have to lead to your acting on the feelings. But the feelings must be taken seriously. See the resources at the end of this chapter for a suicide prevention organization and ways of locating treatment. It *can* get better!

If you are currently in treatment, be sure to tell your counselor about these feelings and work out a plan for what to do if you are in danger of acting on them. Find out who to call and where to go for help after hours. If your counselor does not give you clear answers, seek additional help elsewhere. Your life and the lives of others are at stake.

Self-medication is common. *Self-medication* is the idea that when people have an emotional problem, they may turn to substances to "medicate" themselves (Khantzian 1997). A person with generalized anxiety disorder may use alcohol to relax. A person with depression may use cocaine to feel energy. A person with an eating disorder may use speed to lose weight. That's why it's so important to get help with your co-occurring disorder—if you get help, you may no longer need to use a substance to feel better.

Co-occurring disorders do not go away with abstinence. Some people find that as they get clean from substances, they feel less depressed, anxious, or angry. This is one of the really positive sides of recovery. However, if you have a true co-occurring disorder, it won't go away with abstinence. It needs direct attention and help. The tricky part is that while people are using substances or withdrawing from them, it may look like they have a co-occurring disorder (e.g., depression), but it disappears as they get clean. This means they didn't have a real co-occurring disorder. They had a *substance-induced mental disorder*—what looked like a co-occurring disorder was actually caused by the substance, and goes away when the substance use goes away.

It generally takes four to six weeks of abstinence from all substances to see whether you really have a co-occurring disorder. If the signs persist, you have one; if they go away, you don't. Either way, you can then decide what to do next. If you have a co-occurring disorder, you may need therapy or medication over a period of time. If you don't, good for you—you can just work on maintaining abstinence. However, don't think you have to complete four to six weeks of clean time before you can address your co-occurring problem. It's better to treat it immediately, and if it goes away as you get clean, you can decide later whether to continue the treatment.

A co-occurring disorder is never an excuse to keep using substances. While an emotional disorder is a serious issue that needs attention, it's never an excuse to keep using substances. Indeed, using substances often makes it worse. Cocaine can intensify your anxiety problems, for example. Even if using doesn't make it worse, you're delaying your healing from both the emotional problem and the addiction. It's well known that to fully heal from an emotional problem, you must be clean from substances. Substances distort emotions—either numbing or intensifying them. You want to know the "real you"—not the "false you" on a substance. If substances soothe your emotional difficulties in the short run (e.g., drinking to sleep at night), in the long run they never solve the underlying problem. Sometimes, people with misguided sympathy might say, "If you have depression, it's no wonder you can't recover from addiction. I can understand that you keep using." Wrong! It's all the more important to get clean when you have an emotional problem. It means you need extra-special care and extra-strong focus on recovery from *both* addiction and the emotional disorder.

Be realistic about family members' ability to understand your emotional problem. In a perfect world, you would tell them about your emotional problem and they would support you, being even more kind because now they know how you're suffering. The reality is often different. It may take a long time for them to understand. Your addiction may have caused so many problems that they think you're making excuses. They may have their own emotional problems that they don't want to face—indeed, many emotional problems run in families (Kendler, Davis, and Kessler 1997). It will be important to find people who *do* understand—mental health professionals, other treaters, and support groups of people with similar problems. It's good to show your family members the resources at the end of this chapter to help them learn more about your emotional problem. But stay realistic—it may take them a while, or they may never truly understand. Right now, just focus on helping yourself.

Taking a psychiatric medication is not substance use. Sometimes people hear that taking a psychiatric medication (such as an antidepressant or antianxiety drug) is the same as using a substance. They may hear this from well-meaning people who are truly trying to help them. They may even hear it at AA meetings (even though it's not the official policy of AA). The problem is that it's just not true. First of all, psychiatric medications do not get you "high" when they are taken as prescribed. They simply bring your mood to a normal level. Second, most psychiatric medications are not addictive. Those that are (e.g., benzodiazepines, such as valium, for anxiety) are used cautiously or not at all when someone has an addiction. (Thus, it's very important to tell your doctor your addiction history.) The bottom line is this: taking a psychiatric medication as prescribed, under the supervision of a doctor who understands your history, may be an important part of recovery from emotional problems. There's no "magic bullet"—some disorders are more likely to be helped by medication than others. Usually medication has its best effects when combined with psychotherapy; and it may take some trial and error to identify the medication that works best for you. But psychiatric medication is one of the major advances in the past several decades. There are more of them now and they are safer than before. Thus, you owe it to yourself to at least find out from a doctor whether a medication might help. It will be up to you to decide if you want to take it.

Which came first? That's less important than getting help for both. As in the classic question, "Which came first, the chicken or the egg?", there is sometimes no clear answer to the question of which came first—the addiction or the emotional disorder. Emotional disorders can lead to addiction (e.g., you feel depressed so you use alcohol to feel better), and addiction can lead to emotional disorders (e.g., you use cocaine and develop panic disorder). Or both may arise at the same time—for example, you developed PTSD and substance addiction as a child due to both being abused and being given substances. Even if you do know which came first, by the time you have both, they both need immediate treatment. While it may be helpful at some point to explore how each disorder developed, right now the goal is to get the help for both problems, regardless of which came first (Knowlton 1995; Weiss et al. 1998).

Know that many treatment programs are not yet "up to speed" on dual recovery. You may hear messages that go against what is said here. Someone may say, "AA has been around longer than anything else; don't mess with what works," or, "If you have substance addiction, we can't treat you; we only deal with emotional problems," or, "We've been doing this a long time and know you have to get clean first." Unfortunately these messages are still common. Even though dual recovery is now widely recommended, treatment systems are naturally slower to change. It generally takes ten to twenty years for major shifts to occur. Front-line treaters are there to help, but they may simply be too busy to keep up with all the latest developments.

If you want to read the most up-to-date summary in the addiction field on co-occurring disorders, you can order free from the government the publication *Treatment Improvement Protocol: Assessment and Treatment of Patients with Coexisting Mental Illness and Alcohol and Other Drug Abuse* (CSAT 1994b; see also CSAT in press). These monographs were developed by the government to help improve the quality of treatment in the community. They are based on the agreement of a wide variety of people in the field: experts, researchers, people in recovery, and treaters. You can order free materials on other addiction topics as well (e.g., treatment of addiction in women, rural areas, criminal justice, pregnancy, teens, and gays and lesbians). These materials were written for counselors, but are presented in a clear, concise style. How to order them? See the listing for the National Clearinghouse for Alcohol and Drug Information in the resources section of chapter 1.

Next Steps

So what to do if you want help for your emotional problem? The first step is just to find out more information, keeping an open mind. You don't have to commit to anything. Once you hear more, you can decide what's next. You can choose your own path.

You may feel wary. You may never have sought help before. You may think, "I don't want medication," or "Therapy can't help me." You may have tried to get help in the past and found it didn't work. You may have concerns that someone could force you to stay in treatment or take medication. These are understandable feelings.

It may help to know that, except for a few very extreme situations, your treatment is really in your hands. There are many laws safeguarding your right to be independent. Generally, people can only be forced into treatment when they make a clear and immediate threat to seriously hurt themselves or others physically, or if they are almost completely unable to care for themselves (e.g., they're living without food or clothing). Even under these extreme conditions, you can only be committed to a hospital for a limited amount of time and a judge would have to approve it. For medication, the rules are even more restrictive: in general, you cannot be required to take medication. These extreme conditions are mentioned only because some people never get help out of fear that someone could take away their power. You should talk to a lawyer if you have any concerns and to find out the laws for your state, but overall, don't let these issues prevent you from seeking help.

So how to proceed? Here are some ideas:

+ **Contact any of the resources at the end of this chapter.** All these organizations exist to help people with emotional problems. You can get basic information or ask advice to locate a support group or professional in your community.

+ **Go to the section Seek Support in chapter 6.** It offers suggestions for finding help. If possible, find a mental health professional (e.g., a psychologist, social worker, or psychiatrist) who is trained to understand emotional problems.

+ **Read about others with emotional problems.** Several books are listed at the end of this chapter that may help you understand what you're going through.

It's up to you now. As Horace said, "Dare to be wise; begin!"

☎ Resources

National Institute of Mental Health	800-647-2642 (general number) 800-421-4211 (for a brochure on depression)	www.nimh.nih.gov
American Self-Help Clearinghouse Support groups for mental health	[no website]	www.mentalhelp.net/selfhelp
Substance Abuse and Mental Health Services Administration Mental health referrals	800-789-CMHS	www.mentalhealth.org
National Alliance for the Mentally Ill	800-950-NAMI	www.nami.org
American Foundation for Suicide Prevention	888-333-2377	www.afsp.org
Suicide Prevention Advocacy Network	888-649-1366	www.spansusa.org
National Depressive and Manic Depressive Association	800-826-3632	www.ndmda.org
National Foundation for Depressive Illness	800-239-1265	www.depression.org
National Mental Health Association	800-969-6642	www.nmha.org
Anxiety Disorders Association of America	301-231-9350	www.adaa.org
Panic Disorder Information—National Institute of Mental Health	800-64-PANIC	www.nimh.nih.gov
Anxiety Disorders Information—National Institute of Mental Health	800-8-ANXIETY	www.nimh.nih.gov
Depression After Delivery For postpartum depression	800-944-4PPD	www.depressionafterdelivery.com

Depression Awareness, Recognition and Treatment (DART)— National Institute of Mental Health	800-421-4211	www.nimh.nih.gov/publicat/ depressionmenu.cfm

See also the resources in chapter 3 for information on PTSD, stress, and eating disorders.

What It's Like

It can also be helpful to read what others who have been through an emotional problem say about it. All the books listed are personal accounts of what the problem was like and how the person got help. Many others are available; you can find them at libraries and by searching on the Internet.

+ *Fountain House: Portraits of Lives Reclaimed from Mental Illness* by Mary Flannery and Mark Glickman (about a variety of emotional problems)

+ *Darkness Visible* by William Styron (about depression)

+ *Noonday Demon: An Atlas of Depression* by Andrew Solomon (about depression)

+ *An Unquiet Mind* by Kay Jamison (about bipolar disorder)

+ *Manic by Midnight* by Faye Joy Shannon and Mary Jo Elsasser (about bipolar disorder)

+ *Surviving the Silence: Black Women's Stories of Rape* by Charlotte Pierce-Baker (about rape/PTSD)

+ *After Silence: Rape and My Journey Back* by Nancy Venable Raine (about rape/PTSD)

+ *Sybil* by Flora Rheta Schreiber (about dissociative identity disorder)

+ *Diary of an Eating Disorder: A Mother and Daughter Share Their Healing Journey* by Chelsea Smith and Beverly Runyon (about eating disorder)

+ *The Boy Who Couldn't Stop Washing: The Experience and Treatment of Obsessive Compulsive Disorder* by Judith L. Rapoport (about obsessive-compulsive disorder)

+ *Girl, Interrupted* by Susanna Kaysen (about borderline personality disorder)

PART II

Healing

CHAPTER 5

Ideas on Healing

If life knocks you down seven times, you get up eight.

—Chinese proverb

Healing is about finding a way to move forward. The idea is that *no matter what happens in life,* you can find a healthy way to respond.

Notice the difference between "good coping" and "poor coping." Good coping means you seek solutions that protect you. Poor coping means you respond destructively—with addictive behavior or other dangerous action, or just by doing nothing at all. Tough times happen to everyone. But no matter how awful a time, there's a way to respond well and a way that drags you down further. "No situation is so bad that I can't make it worse by the way I handle it," Manter du Wors wrote (1992). The flip side is that no situation is so bad that you can't make it better by handling it well. Handling it well builds internal strength and self-respect.

Women with addiction have less healthy coping than those who are not addicted. This has been found over and over in research (Cisler and Nawrocki 1998; Michels et al. 1999). Thus, to heal, they need to learn how to cope better. This second half of the book explores ways to do that.

There are four ways of coping with life: through *people, actions, beliefs,* and *feelings.* Each is a different way of engaging with the world, a different type of knowledge. *Healing through people* means, for example, talking honestly, accepting help, choosing friends, and resolving conflicts. It's about viewing people as an important part of your life. *Healing through actions* means concrete steps, such as taking care of your body, controlling harmful impulses, and moving forward despite fear. It's about "voting with your feet"—the bottom line is how you act. *Healing through beliefs* is you within your own mind: how you talk to yourself, what you believe in, listening to your different sides. *Healing through feelings* is using feelings (both good and bad) as a tool to guide you: mourning losses, finding acceptance, and soothing yourself, for example. It's honoring that all feelings are there for a reason.

The next four chapters will offer growth exercises in each of these areas. With addiction, your life became narrow. Now the goal is to expand. You can "play" with the exercises—doing them in any order, skipping around to what interests you. You may find you do some just once, others many times. If there are some you don't like, you can just let those go.

Keys to Healing

Across the four domains are several broad principles of recovery. If you want, put a star next to those below you agree with. Put a question mark next to those you don't understand. If you disagree with some, leave them alone.

+ **Just do the best next step.** It's "like driving a car at night. You can see only as far as your headlights, but you can make the whole trip that way" (E. L. Doctorow, in Lamott 1994, 18). The beauty of this is that you don't have to plan it all out or even to believe it'll work. As long as you're choosing, right this moment, to do the best you can with what's in front of you, eventually you'll arrive. One next step after another.

✦ **It's okay if it feels all wrong.** You may believe that if you're doing recovery right, it'll feel right. But at times it feels all wrong. You think, "I still want to use," "I'm getting more depressed as I get clean," or "I'm confused." These thoughts are normal in early recovery. The goal is just to hang in there, no matter what. Over time, an inner sense of clarity will emerge. Like the cocoon that conceals a butterfly, recovery may not look beautiful as it develops.

✦ **It's usually many small things rather than one big thing.** Some people have a flash of insight, like lightning, and never use again. The philosopher William James described this as a conversion experience a century ago, and it became the basis of the AA movement (James 1902/1958). It may feel religious, like divine intervention. But for many other people, healing doesn't work this way. It's just the day in and day out little things: eating a meal, taking a walk to calm down, distracting yourself to ride out a craving, getting sleep, showing up at treatment. They may not seem big or magical, but they work. Eventually you create an upward spiral of growth, rather than the downward spiral of addiction.

✦ **You don't have to go far to heal.** Everything is right around you. Sometimes people delay the healing process because they believe they must create ideal conditions before they begin. They want to get themselves ready, they want to find just the right program, they want to relocate to another part of the country. But really, it's all right where you are, right now. You can throw out your stash of substances, you can read about addiction, you can find self-help groups, you can get on the Internet, you can try new coping skills. Delay never helps addiction.

✦ **What seems bad may end up good.** A common theme in recovery is that what at first seemed bad became a turning point. People who were forced into treatment often say this launched their recovery process, though at first they were angry and bitter. All the stories of "hitting bottom" are about losses that ultimately turned people's lives around—losing a job, children, home, or partner. At your darkest moments, you may feel certain that life is hopeless. But you can use any experience to steer toward recovery. In the end, those dark moments may save you. Judgments of "good" and "bad" can only be clear with the benefit of time—looking back, from the perspective of sobriety.

✦ **It is within you to heal.** You're human and thus have the potential to grow. Everyone does, no matter how long they've been addicted. Healing is as natural a process as physical growth. It's a deep reservoir you can tap into at any point. The philosopher Plato observed that knowledge is within, waiting to be discovered. As you try new ways, you discover who you really are.

✦ **Try.** Good coping is active—it's about trying. Poor coping is passive—it's waiting, doing nothing, hoping it'll all work out somehow. And here's the big trick: you can start *anywhere*. Good coping is not about choosing the right thing or The Solution or even the same thing over and over. It's just "do something, anything." As long as the activity promotes healing, it counts. Go with your moods and preferences. One day it may help to listen to soothing music, another day to clean your house, another day to go to a self-help meeting.

✦ **Hang on to both sides.** In recovery, you're continually balancing opposites: letting yourself feel your deepest feelings and, at other times, moving away from them when they're too intense or destructive; focusing on your needs and seeing the needs of others; working hard and taking rest. Balancing these opposites, learning to move in and out of them at will, represents real growth. The key is not to believe that only one side is the right way. Both are needed at different times, just as a carpenter uses different tools depending on the job.

✦ **Be curious about yourself.** Healing from addiction means getting to know yourself. Amid the haze of a substance is a person you come to see more and more clearly. Be curious about who she is. Treat her as you would a new friend: try to understand her, see what she likes and dislikes. As you try new ways of coping, see how she reacts—what works and what doesn't. Being curious, rather than judgmental, keeps you open to learning.

✦ **Tell the truth**. When you tell the truth, you open a door. You may cringe when you see how low you've sunk, who you've hurt, what you've allowed your life to become. But if you can face what you know, you can get beyond it. The very definition of mental illness is avoiding reality, living in illusion. No matter how painful the truth, it always leads to something good over time.

✦ **Listen to what you want.** Using a substance is usually a misguided attempt to feel good—to feel energy, thrills, connection, calm, freedom. You're not wrong for wanting these. But the task is getting them without a substance. "Anything you can do with drugs you can do without drugs," William Burroughs said. Listen closely to your needs and find new ways to gratify them. Many women long ago gave up listening to their needs to focus on others. Now can be a time to return to your needs too.

✦ **Above all, be kind.** Just as a child does better in response to praise, noticing what you are doing right and being gentle with yourself will sustain you through the rough patches. But being kind never means letting yourself off easy—indeed, the opposite. Recovery is about asking the best of yourself and sticking to your commitments, no matter what. But you're more likely to achieve these with strong encouragement and reassurance. It's easy to yell at yourself, put yourself down, call yourself names. Kindness is harder, but more true.

Once you learn to cope with life without substances, no one can take that away. They might be able to take material possessions—your money or house perhaps—but they can't take away that inner strength once you've built it within. It's like learning to read: when you know it, you have it forever. The writer Anne Lamott describes this truth in a visit to her pastor:

I said that I was all over the place, up and down, scattered, high, withdrawing, lost, and in the midst of it all trying to find some elusive sense of serenity.

"The world can't give us serenity," he said. "The world can't give us peace. We can only find it in our hearts."

"I hate that," I said.

"I know. But the good news is that by the same token, the world can't take it away." (1994, 221)

An Example of Coping

Imagine the following scene: Jessie got the news that her only sister died suddenly in a car accident. She's devastated. They were so close. Their children played together, and the two families vacationed at the beach each summer. Her whole life will be different now. She always imagined they would go through life side by side, comparing notes along the way. Now she's alone.

Poor coping. Jessie's in shock. She's depressed and feels nothing will ever be the same. She tries to get up and do things—work, shop, clean, go to the movies—but nothing feels right. She's never dealt with the death of someone close to her before, and she truly believes she'll never get over it. She can't cry and feels guilty about that. Her husband tries to talk to her, but she feels no one will understand. She isolates more and more. She starts drinking after five years sober. She's hiding bottles in the basement again. This goes on for several months and she knows it's not good, but she can't stop. She feels awful. She has fleeting thoughts of suicide.

How did Jessie cope? She . . .

- Isolated

- Drank

- Kept secrets

- Told herself no one would understand

- Let a bad situation continue

- Didn't seek help

- Told herself she'd never get over it

- Began thinking of suicide

Good coping. Jessie knows she's in deeper than she can handle. She sees her urges to drink and inability to cry as signs that she needs help. She finds a local grief support group, and goes to the library to read about grieving. She learns that it's not unusual to have a delayed reaction, and that she can just accept whatever feelings come up or don't come up. She confides to the group that she felt disloyal to her sister by not crying. She talks about feeling that she can't go on, and they share their stories of heartache. She makes efforts to do things that she knows her sister would have liked—helping out with her kids, creating a garden to remember her by, giving to her sister's favorite charity. She tells her husband about her urges to drink. He encourages her to go to more AA meetings. Over many months, she's eventually able to cry. It's horribly painful, but she knows she needs to go through the feelings. Slowly, the sadness is replaced by more of her old self. She'll never forget her sister, but she knows her sister would want her to live fully and joyfully.

How did Jessie cope? She . . .

+ Saw danger signs in herself

+ Learned how others cope with grief

+ Found a support group

+ Confided in people

+ Accepted her own pace

+ Attended more AA meetings

+ Actively did things that her sister would have liked

+ Let herself cry

Do you see the difference? It's the same situation, but in one case, Jessie responds in ways that make her life worse. In the other, she's able to move toward healing. That's the essence of what we'll be exploring in the rest of the book—how to choose wisely, in ways that nurture rather than destroy you.

CHAPTER 6

Healing Through Relationships

Good relationships are like gold—they enrich your life. To feel understanding, belonging, and love are some of the deepest needs people have.

But relationships can also bring misery. Sometimes they're far worse than being alone. Domestic violence, family abuse, and people betraying your confidence or undermining your efforts—all of these can drag you down.

At the low point of an addiction, your most important relationship is usually your substance. Caroline Knapp describes it as a love story: "It's about passion, sensual pleasure, deep pulls, lust, fears, yearning hungers. It's about needs so strong they're crippling" (1997, 7).

Thus, recovery almost always involves relationship building—replacing your addiction with real relationships. Similarly, finding sober friends to replace addicted friends is part of the work. Many people fear they can't connect with others without being intoxicated—they believe they won't be fun, relaxed, or sexy enough.

This chapter offers four relationship skills:

- Tell a secret
- Share responsibility
- Become friends with women
- Seek support

The paradox is that working on your relationships means working on yourself above all. Sometimes people believe that it's about trying to change others. But you are more likely to succeed if you turn the spotlight on yourself. As you grow, you'll find that other people will grow too. As you develop better relationship skills, you'll naturally attract better people into your life.

Most people want love more than anything else. Women especially rely on relationships and use them as a way of understanding the world (Jordan et al. 1991). This can be a real strength, allowing them to build bonds of family and community. Unfortunately, the flip side is that many women stay in bad relationships just to feel some semblance of love. They may be so afraid of being alone or abandoned that they'll give up their very self to stay part of a couple, for example. The relationship skills in this chapter are thus designed to build healthy relationships and to let go of unhealthy ones. Intimacy—not just companionship—is the goal.

Growth Exercise: *Tell a Secret*

One of the best ways to build close relationships is to share your innermost thoughts. This is true for everyone, but if you have an addiction, you may be hiding a lot from people. Women with addiction are known to carry even more shame and guilt than addicted men, due to society's more negative views of addicted women. You may feel that you're carrying a heavy burden that you alone know. You may feel alienated from people, or just bad about yourself.

Breaking the silence can bring more intimacy. The goal is to feel that you don't have to hide anything—that one or more people in your life know the real you. It's said that "misery shared is misery halved." By sharing secrets, you move toward your genuine self, away from a false self. It's freeing, like your soul taking flight.

What are examples of secrets?

- "There are things I did while high that I'm very ashamed of."
- "I may look strong, but inside I'm in a lot of pain."
- "I used a lot more than I let on."
- "I feel angry with you; it's hard for me to tell you that."
- "I have thoughts of hurting myself."
- "I feel I'm not as smart or popular as other people."

How?

The idea is to tell a secret in a way that is most likely to be successful. Because telling a secret makes one feel so vulnerable, it can be devastating to open your heart if the other person doesn't understand—or worse, is critical or rejecting. It's important to do this exercise carefully.

Step I: Prepare

1. **Choose a secret that really matters;** one you haven't ever told anyone, or perhaps one that you've been wanting to reveal to a particular person. Remember, the more vulnerable the secret makes you, the more closeness you gain. Write a few words here that will remind you what it is. You don't have to write it out fully as you may not want to have it down on paper. Example: "1997—what I did that summer when I had the house to myself."

---

2. **Write down who you'll tell.** Be sure to pick someone you think will be supportive and kind. You could try your therapist or sponsor, or anyone else in your life that you feel can "hear" you.

---

3. **Be clear on what you want.** For example, "I want you to just listen and not judge me for it," or, "I'd like you to tell me I'm not a horrible person," or, "I want to know that you won't ever tell anyone what I'm about to say."

_____

_____

_____

4. **Create a plan that is likely to work.** This means not "spilling" your secret casually or randomly. That isn't fair to you or the other person. Make sure to pick a good time and place (but don't delay forever!). You might say, "I'd like to tell you something very personal that I haven't told anyone. Is that okay? Is this a good time?" Rehearse it in your mind in advance. If possible, create a backup plan for what you'll do if the conversation doesn't go well (how you'll soothe yourself and seek support).

_____

_____

_____

5. **How difficult will it be for you to tell your secret?**

0	1	2	3
Not at all difficult	A little difficult	Moderately difficult	Extremely difficult

Know that telling a secret feels difficult; you may feel embarrassed, weak, or childlike. That's the nature of secrets. But it's extremely freeing once you've done it. (If you circled "0," consider choosing a harder secret; otherwise you may not get much out of this exercise.)

6. **After sharing your secret, fill out the next section.**

Step II: Reflect

Write down what happened, how it felt, what you gained, any surprises, and other thoughts.

_____

_____

_____

_____

Growth Exercise: *Share Responsibility*

Many women are overly apologetic and take too much of the blame in relationship conflicts. They feel they're at fault whenever things go wrong. They feel they always need to defer to the other person. Other women do the opposite. They view conflicts as all the other person's fault. And, if you're like most people, you may swing to both extremes, sometimes taking too much responsibility, sometimes too little.

Addiction may increase these tendencies. It intensifies your emotions and leaves you less able to see relationship problems clearly. Also, addiction prevents emotional growth. You stay stuck at a younger stage, so these relationship patterns may persist longer than they otherwise would have.

This growth exercise is about getting a balanced view. It's about learning to see both people's responsibility in a conflict. All relationship problems *between adults* require two people—if just one person is the problem, there won't be a conflict. For example, if someone is criticizing you, you have many possible responses. You can agree, disagree, walk away, discuss the criticism, request that the person talk to you in a different manner, etc. There are many ways you could react. If you take into account both your point of view and the other person's, there likely won't be a problem. If you see only one person's side, there likely will be a problem. For example, if you "own" just your point of view, you may too easily dismiss the other person's concerns and the situation can escalate into a power struggle. If you "own" just the other person's point of view, you may give in too easily and disregard your needs. Thus, the goal is balance—seeing both sides clearly.

Keep in mind that these ideas apply only to adults. Children will naturally react in ways that are immature. They also have less power than adults, so must be related to differently.

How?

It can help to imagine a chart that lets you visualize how much you're taking on in a conflict. Then you can try to balance it out, aiming to share responsibility for what went wrong. It's like the children's story of Goldilocks. She finds three chairs: one is too big, one is too little, and the last one is just right.

An example of a "responsibility chart" follows, along with some ideas about how to share responsibility. Then you can take one of your current relationship conflicts and try the exercise.

Example

Pat and Andrea are friends. Andrea is upset with Pat, saying, "I can't believe you betrayed my confidence. When I told you last week I was quitting my job, you weren't supposed to go and tell the world. Now a whole bunch of people know. How could you do this to me?" In fact, Pat did tell several people, but she didn't know that Andrea wanted the information kept confidential.

If Pat takes *too much* responsibility, she says to Andrea, "I'm so sorry—I can't believe I did that. I don't blame you for being mad. I won't do it again." Her chart will look like this:

Pat's responsibility	Andrea's responsibility

If Pat takes *too little* responsibility, she says to Andrea, "Well, you never told me not to tell anyone. It's not right to blame me. I can't believe you'd talk to me this way." Her chart will look like this:

Pat's responsibility	Andrea's responsibility

So the goal for Pat will be to share responsibility. It's best to assume in relationships that both people contribute to the problems that come up. If she takes a balanced view, she might say to Andrea, "I understand you're upset—I see now that you wanted the information kept private. I hope you know that I wouldn't betray your confidence intentionally. I didn't know that you wanted it kept private. How about if next time I'll ask you if it's confidential, and could you also try to let me know that? I don't want this to ever happen again." Her chart might look like this:

Pat's responsibility	Andrea's responsibility

A few suggestions for working on this topic are as follows:

✦ You don't need to focus on exactly how much each person was responsible. Whether it was 50–50, 60–40, or even 80–20, that's not the point. You may certainly have your view on this. But the goal is just to see that both people contribute to a conflict. There is always some way in which each person can do better to improve the relationship.

✦ Notice how it feels to share responsibility. Doesn't it seem more hopeful? It means you're both in this together. You can feel closer to the other person, because you realize that everyone makes relationship mistakes and everyone can do better.

✦ When you share responsibility, you develop more compassion. You move beyond just one point of view. It takes more effort to see both sides, but it gives you more insight.

✦ What to do if the other person isn't willing to accept any responsibility? If this is a repeated problem (not just a onetime event), you may need to let the relationship go. See the growth exercise Accept in chapter 9.

Your Turn

Now it's your turn. Describe a current relationship problem three ways: where you take too much responsibility; where you take too little responsibility; and finally, balanced responsibility.

1. Describe a current relationship problem with you taking *too much* responsibility.

_____

_____

_____

_____

| Your responsibility | The other person's reponsibility |

2. Describe the same relationship problem with you taking *too little* responsibility.

_____

_____

_____

_____

| Your responsibility | The other person's responsibility |

3. Now describe the same current relationship problem with you and the other person *sharing* responsibility.

_____

_____

_____

_____

| Your responsibility | The other person's responsibility |

Growth Exercise: *Become Friends with Women*

It would seem that women who share a common problem such as addiction would be drawn to supporting each other. Too often, though, they focus just on men, or they distrust other women. Many have no women friends (Lichtenstein 1997).

How many women do you have as friends? How close are you to them? If you haven't cultivated women as friends, you may want to look more closely at why. Many women view other women negatively. They may not even be fully aware of it. But their behavior says it all: they "blow off" their women friends when a man comes into their life, they treat women less well than men, they listen more to men, they defer more to men. They're also more critical of women: they think less of a woman who isn't married or doesn't have children, but they don't do this with men. They judge women more on appearance and on whether they fit in. Heterosexual women may be especially prone to these biases, but other women may have them as well.

When women behave in these ways, they're not trying to be disrespectful. They likely grew up absorbing the message that men are more valuable than women (e.g., "You're nothing without a man"). They also may project onto other women their own worst feelings about themselves. This means that if you dislike yourself, you come to dislike other women—you see yourself in them. Or you may not want to associate with them because you secretly look down on them, believing they're "weak" or "too emotional," for example. Some women view other women mostly as competition in the quest for a man, rather than seeing them as people in their own right. When you think of how recently women obtained basic equality in society, these views are not surprising. It takes a long time for attitudes to shift.

Why are women important for your recovery? First, it's a statement of how you view yourself. If you value other women, you're saying that you value yourself. Second, friendships are an important source of support. While romantic relationships may be exciting, they are prone to breakups, conflict, and instability. If you can build a network of steady friends, your recovery is on more solid footing. You can enjoy men friends, but it's important to have women friends too.

Women can understand some aspects of your experience better, just because they're women. This doesn't mean all women will understand you all the time, but it does mean they faced many of the same issues you have. Women are more likely to be the primary caretaker of children, to be single parents, to be abandoned by a partner once they become addicted, to be paid less than men, to have less power in the workplace, to be abused as children, and to be sexually harassed. These are simply facts. You need people who can understand you. Many women say that once they develop friendships with women, they are their best friends, the ones they can talk to about anything. Even if you're someone who prefers men, you can learn to draw from this incredible source for at least some of your friendship needs.

How?

This exercise encourages you to notice your deep-down views of women, and then helps you to find more women friends.

Step I: Become Aware of Your Views of Women

1. **How many women friends do you have?** Include only those you see or talk to at least once every three months (and not just at work or AA, for example, but because you make the effort to stay in touch outside of organized meetings).
   _____

2. **When you think of women, which of these ideas pop into mind?**
   - ☐ Weak
   - ☐ Too emotional
   - ☐ No ethics
   - ☐ Competitive about men
   - ☐ No sense of humor
   - ☐ Less interesting than men
   - ☐ Too focused on their looks
   - ☐ Talk too much
   - ☐ Don't play fair
   - ☐ Achieve less than men
   - ☐ Nice to your face, but talk behind your back
   - ☐ Too focused on their kids
   - ☐ Bad drivers
   - ☐ Other negative view: _____

How many did you check off above? _____
   - ☐ Loyal
   - ☐ Supportive
   - ☐ Strong
   - ☐ Caring
   - ☐ Responsible
   - ☐ High-achieving
   - ☐ Valued in society
   - ☐ Talented
   - ☐ Insightful
   - ☐ Good at sports
   - ☐ Good at relationships
   - ☐ Open and honest
   - ☐ Stable

☐ Fun

☐ Other positive view: _____

How many did you check off in this second section? _____

If you want, you can also do some writing. How do you feel about having women friends? How important are they to you? Do you treat them as well as men? Do you have secret negative judgments of them?

_____

_____

_____

_____

_____

What do you get from this exercise? Hopefully, you see your views of women more clearly. It's okay to own your negative judgments. That's the starting point for developing real friendships with women. If you can be honest, you can move beyond where you are now.

Hopefully, too, you hear the underlying message: it's important to respect women—both yourself and others. People are people, and you will naturally like some more than others. But if you have a gender bias, you may want to strive for a more sophisticated view—evaluating individuals rather than writing off women in general. There are good women out there, just as there are good men.

Step II: Find Women Friends

As they say, "Where there's a will there's a way." If you decide you want to become friends with women, you will start finding opportunities all around you. Here are some suggestions:

✦ **Find role models of strong women.** Notice women leaders in your community, at work, and in the media. Develop a picture in your mind of women who are strong and good? *Can you think of any?*

_____

_____

✦ **Cultivate relationships with women.** Look around to find women you like, and try to really focus on them—make the extra effort to start a conversation and stay in touch. *Can you think of any?*

_____

_____

✦ **Strive to keep your friendships with women steady.** Even if men drift in and out of your life, stay anchored to your women friends. Keep up contact no matter what else is going on. *Can you think of ways to do this?*

_____

_____

✦ **Notice how you react toward women versus toward men.** Keep watching your own thoughts and behavior. Do you do more for men? Do you judge them differently? It's been said that "the best way to have a friend is to be a friend." Act toward women in ways that you want to be treated. *Can you think of ways to do this?*

_____

_____

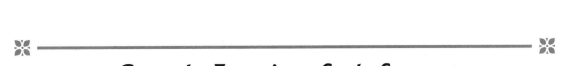

Growth Exercise: *Seek Support*

The two simple words "seek support" can bridge the distance between addiction and recovery. Seeking support means finding help anywhere you can—family and friends, treatment, self-help, reading, calling 800 numbers—truly, whatever you can grasp onto to make the journey easier.

When you reach out, you open yourself up to the wisdom of others. You replace addictive relationships with real relationships. Seeking help is especially important for women, who are known to get less support for recovery, seek help later than men, and underutilize treatment resources (Blume 1998; Walitzer and Connors 1997).

If you're isolated or grew up not being able to trust the people around you, it may feel scary to ask for help. If you're always the strong, competent one, you may find it hard to let your guard down and let others in. Even if you want support you may not know how to find it.

It's important to choose your helpers carefully. You may find some wonderful helpers and others who give you a queasy feeling. Learn to trust your gut. Good help feels good. Bad help feels confusing, makes you feel "put down," or may feel like a battle. One study of women in treatment showed that 42 percent reported invalidating, unskilled, or sexually harassing professionals (Schellenberg 1998). Some treaters are burned out with low salaries, increased paperwork, and large caseloads

(Rosenheck 1999). Some are trained to handle emotional problems (such as depression and PTSD), while others aren't. There is good help out there, but you may need to search for a while.

Also, don't rely on simple judgments. The amount of money charged, the person's degree (e.g., Ph.D. versus B.A.), number of years of experience, and gender, for example, have all been found not to make a difference in how helpful a treater is. One common myth is that treaters who are in recovery are better than those who aren't, but this isn't true; over fifty studies show no difference. Treaters *do* differ greatly in their ability to achieve good results with clients, but it's a more subtle set of qualities that distinguish the best from the worst (McLellan et al. 1988; Najavits, Crits-Christoph, and Dierberger 2000).

Whatever help you select, you can always change your mind later. Make your best guess and see where it leads. You may find that your needs change over time—what works now may feel outdated later. As discussed in chapter 2, people may express strong opinions. They may tell you there's just one way or predict that your future is grim unless you do what they did. But there are many paths. The Fletcher study of 222 people who succeeded in recovery showed a broad range: some used AA, some didn't. Some relied on professionals, others didn't (2001). Some did it a day at a time, others made a commitment for life. Some hit bottom, others caught the problem early. Some used spirituality, some didn't. In short, the path to healing means listening very closely to what *you* need.

If, however, you find yourself revolving through a large number of programs or sponsors, with no one being "good enough," you may need to look within. It's one thing to shop around until you find someone you click with; but if literally nothing works, most likely you need to pick something and stick with it long enough to let the magic happen. Some people dart from one program to another in a frenzied attempt to do absolutely anything except look at themselves. The famous "geographic cure" doesn't work either (e.g., "If I move out West, it'll all come together"). You'll still be you once you get there; only the weather will be different. One important exception: if you are surrounded by addicted people or live in a drug-infested community, moving away can help.

It's a sign of strength to reach out for support. It means you can hear and be heard, you can see and be seen. Going through life alone is like being a ghost—no one knows you. Support gives you a boost. It makes things easier, more stable. It gives you people to bounce ideas off of. It lets you vent feelings. It makes you see that other people have problems too, and that other people also find a way out. It's not that you can't do recovery alone, but it's harder. And for severe addictions, the odds are stacked against you unless you get help.

If some people aren't helpful, let them go. Don't try to fix them or demand that they be what you need. That's a big job, and they have to want to change. Right now, focus on you. Be like a mouse in a maze: if you hit a dead end, turn around and try another route. If you obsess about someone who's disappointing you, it's a distraction from bigger issues.

Some women do best in programs designed for women. Women's AA groups, reinterpretations of the 12 steps for women (Covington 1994; Kasl 1992), self-help groups such as Women for Sobriety, and women-and-children programs may make it easier for you to connect. Research shows these are helpful (Kaskutas 1996; Killeen and Brady 2000), but the jury's still out on whether, overall, women need gender-specific programs (Blume 1998). Again, trust your instincts. One point is clear, however: the longer you stay in treatment, the better you're likely to do (Simpson et al. 1997).

Finally, know that simply seeking information on addiction can make a big difference. A book or just a phrase at the right time can change your life. Reading self-help books, getting on the Internet, and talking to people may seem basic, but they can steer you where you need to go. Such resources are often undervalued, but they are free and quick. The technological revolution offers a wealth of information that wasn't available to people in recovery thirty years ago. Whether you are rich or poor, urban or rural, you can tap into that knowledge base. You can also seek support on all sorts of problems, in addition to addiction, such as stress, depression, love addiction, eating disorders, domestic violence, and gambling. There are resources out there for any problem you may have.

How?

To create more support in your life, there are two steps. The first is to explore what kind of support you might want. The second is to find ways to make it happen.

Step I: Choose Support

What support might work best for you? Check off any that appeal to you. This isn't about what others say or about doing something you don't believe in. Listen to yourself closely and decide, just for right now, what you need. You can change your mind later. *Note: You can also use this list to explore help your child or partner might need if they have an addiction or emotional problem.*

☐ *Individual therapy* (talking to a professional one-on-one about your problems)

☐ *Group therapy* (a professionally led group of people with similar problems)

☐ *Self-help groups* (free peer-led)

☐ *Medication* (for addiction and/or emotional problems)

☐ *Alternative treatments* (such as acupuncture or meditation)

☐ *Skills training* (such as parenting or relationship skills)

☐ *Job training* (to change careers)

☐ *Day treatment* (a half-day or all-day program to get intensive help with addiction or mental health)

☐ *Self-help books* (you can pick any topics that are important to you)

☐ *Sober housing* (a house shared by people committed to abstinence)

☐ *Hospitalization* (around-the-clock care for severe problems)

☐ *Residential programs* (communities dedicated to recovery)

☐ *Religious affiliation* (a church, temple, mosque, or other spiritually-based center)

☐ *School* (take a class to learn more about the type of problem you have)

☐ *Evaluation* (get a professional opinion on what kind of help you need)

☐ *Couples or family therapy* (to sort out intimate relationship problems)

☐ *Domestic violence counseling* (confidential help on what to do if someone is abusing you)

☐ *Housing* (to move or obtain shelter if you are homeless)

☐ *Hotline* (a free number you can call to talk when you're feeling upset)

☐ *Crisis counseling* (immediate assistance if you feel in danger of hurting yourself or others)

☐ *Case management* (someone to help you navigate treatment systems)

☐ *Referral line* (800 numbers to obtain a referral into treatment)

☐ *National resources* (800 numbers on particular problem areas)

☐ *Internet* (online help, such as Web sites and chat rooms for recovery discussions, expert advice, and information)

☐ Other: _____

☐ Other: _____

Step II: Locate Support

There are many ways to find help. You may need to persist to obtain high-quality services or to overcome limitations such as insurance or location. Check off any ways that might work for you.

☐ Contact one or more of the resources (800 numbers) listed in previous chapters of this book.

☐ Call your insurance company and ask for a list of treatment providers.

☐ Ask people you know for recommendations.

☐ Look in the Yellow Pages under headings such as "Addiction," "Subtance Abuse," "Counseling," "Mental Health," "Psychotherapy," "Social Services," or "Clinics." You can also order a copy of the Human Services Yellow Pages from your local telephone company; this is a specialized guide that focuses just on treatment.

☐ Call a local hospital or clinic and ask how to obtain treatment.

☐ Call your local community mental health center.

☐ Go to a self-help meeting; you can ask people there for further ideas.

☐ Ask your medical doctor for a referral.

☐ Search the Internet (public libraries often provide free computer access).

☐ Go to a library and ask the reference librarian to help you identify resources.

☐ Call 411 (information) to get local hotline or crisis-counseling information.

☐ Call a religious organization (many provide or refer people to treatment).

☐ Look at the resource lists in various self-help books.

☐ Look in your local newspaper, which may list support groups.

☐ Other: _____

☐ Other: _____

Self-Awareness Summary

You can use this as a guide to remember the skills you want to keep learning.

How much do you *currently* use these coping skills?

	Not at all	A little	Moderately	Extremely
Tell a secret	0	1	2	3
Share responsibility	0	1	2	3
Become friends with women	0	1	2	3
Seek support	0	1	2	3

How helpful would it be for you to use these coping skills *more*?

	Not at all helpful	A little helpful	Moderately helpful	Extremely helpful
Tell a secret	0	1	2	3
Share responsibility	0	1	2	3
Become friends with women	0	1	2	3
Seek support	0	1	2	3

CHAPTER 7

Healing Through Beliefs

Life presents the question and we give the answer, it's been said. No matter what happens, there are many ways to respond. One person sees a storm on the horizon and thinks, "Isn't nature awesome?"; another thinks, "A storm: just like my life—full of cold misery." Everything is about the *meaning* you give it.

One of the great moments in recovery is when you see that you can *choose* how you think. You can choose whether to view a tough time as a failure or an opportunity. You can choose whether to view your life as valuable or cheap.

Indeed, a whole branch of therapy, cognitive therapy, is devoted to helping people change their thought patterns (Beck et al. 1993). A whole branch of self-help, SMART Recovery, focuses on changing addictive thinking. Whatever words are used—cognitive restructuring, changing your belief system, creating meaning, or self-talk—the gist is the same. It's how you talk to yourself, your internal voice, that can make all the difference.

This chapter provides four growth exercises:

❉ Listen to that small, quiet voice

❉ Ask questions

❉ Create an ideal to live for

❉ Rethink

Each offers a unique angle on a common theme: by changing your beliefs, you can change your reality. In the words of Marcus Aurelius, "Our life is what our thoughts make it."

Growth Exercise:
Listen to That Small, Quiet Voice

In each person there's a "small, quiet voice"—the one that tells you what you know is right. It's called "small and quiet" because it's so easily drowned out by the much louder noises around it—the voice in your head that says "just one won't hurt," the friend offering you a drink at the holiday party.

The small, quiet voice is the one that chooses self-respect. It's the one that knows that what is easiest and feels so right this minute may feel awful later on. It's the one that tells you what you don't want to hear. Like that rare friend who tells you the truth, it's the voice that says, "Just one *will* hurt," "You've been down this road before," and "You know you can't stop."

If you choose to, it's very easy to ignore that small voice. You can overpower it, talk over it, push it away. You can call it stupid. You can tell yourself it's not really there. But it always is there. It's like a heartbeat, steady and present all the time, but so soft that you don't notice it unless you decide to.

This growth exercise is about choosing to hear that small, quiet voice. It asks you to let that voice grow larger, to own that it is there for a reason and that your recovery depends on listening to it.

How?

Here's an example. After that, try the exercise yourself.

Example

You are at dinner in a beautiful restaurant. Everything is great—the food, the service, the décor. The only thing missing is a glass of wine. You're craving the swirl in the glass, the warm calm that gently spreads through your body. You can't stop thinking about it.

What does that small, quiet voice say? "You need to get your mind off drinking. You know where this leads. You'll be throwing it all away if you have that glass of wine. You can pretend not to see it, but you know the truth. Imagine tomorrow and next week. You're a good person who's hurting. You feel deprived. You can get through this. Just enjoy the meal without a drink. You're lucky to be in this nice setting. Don't ruin it."

Your Turn

Now it's your turn. For each situation below, write out what your "small, quiet voice" would say.

1. You're depressed. You wonder, "What's the point of it all? Why bother fighting every day, when nothing seems to change?" You think there's something wrong with you. You want to get high and escape. *What does your small, quiet voice say?*

_____

_____

_____

2. You and your partner have the best sex when you're stoned. It's your anniversary and you want to get high. Anniversaries happen only once a year.... *What does your small, quiet voice say?*

_____

_____

_____

3. Your kids are driving you nuts, your car needs a repair, you don't have enough money, you feel behind in your work. You want to take some pills to get some space—to just calm down. *What does your small, quiet voice say?*

____

____

____

What else do you want to notice about your small, quiet voice? How can you make it larger?

____

____

____

Growth Exercise: *Ask Questions*

Everyone gets stuck sometimes. You're in a dark place, and it feels so very real—as if it's all you've ever known and ever will know. Everything seems to have gone wrong; you can't see a way out. You may feel trapped, and you can't even think straight anymore.

When you're in this place, your mind has become rigid and narrow. There are always choices in life, but you can't see them. This growth exercise is about ways you can shake your mind loose and get flexible in your thinking. It's about learning to have a conversation with yourself that leads you out of the woods, into the light. You ask yourself bold questions and then answer them. Questioning has long been a way that people use to get unstuck. It's used as a method in philosophy, and it's the primary way that therapy works: your therapist asks you questions to help you see things in a new way. In all fields, new knowledge starts from asking good questions.

There's a real art to asking good questions. (Indeed, good questions are really statements—they "know" something.) As kids, we question everything, but as we get older, we think in ruts—same old, same old. You have to train your mind to not just accept your automatic way of thinking, but to wake up. It's about saying, "Life is rich and varied—it has limitless possibilities. I can discover new ways of looking at the world. I can challenge myself to think creatively." When everyone else said the earth was flat, Columbus alone said, "Maybe it's round." It takes guts to go against what you (or others) have been thinking for a long time. It takes courage and will.

When you learn to do it, it feels good. It feels right, because we know that no one has all the answers. Life is about constant learning. There are many ways to learn: you can read books, talk to people, visit new places, even just browse through a magazine you haven't read before. All of these give you a glimpse into a new reality. There are always treasures to uncover.

How?

Step 1: Create Questions

The idea here is to challenge yourself with provocative questions, to break out of your usual thought patterns. It's like shaking the cobwebs and dust from your mind—doing some mental spring cleaning. Circle any below that you like, and make up your own.

✦ What's Plan B, if Plan A doesn't work?

✦ Which way has integrity?

✦ What's missing in this picture?

✦ What's the "message" I hear?

✦ What if I were just as important as anyone else?

✦ In the end, what matters most?

✦ How can I protect myself?

✦ What are my actions saying?

✦ What am I trying to push away?

✦ Is there anyone who can help me?

✦ How can I be there for myself?

✦ Is there an image that can guide me?

✦ What can I do, no matter how imperfect?

✦ What happened in my past that led me here?

✦ What's a real gift I give myself?

✦ If I liked myself, what would I do?

✦ How do I really feel?

✦ Where's the balance?

✦ Are there different sides of myself that I need to hear?

✦ What is safest for me?

✦ Your question: _____

✦ Your question: _____

✦ Your question: _____

Step II: Answer Your Questions

Read the example, then try it for yourself. Note that sometimes you may need to ask yourself more than one question to make it work.

Example

You were three months clean from substances. Yesterday you slipped. You wake up thinking, "I can't do it. I'm not strong enough." *What can you ask yourself to see it in a new way?*

Question: I would ask myself, "What kind of help do I need?"
Answer: I would answer by saying, "I see now that I can't do it alone. I need people to show me the way. This slip can be just a bump in the road—I don't have to let it become a full-blown disaster. If I listen to what this slip is telling me, it's saying I need help. This problem won't go away on its own. Three months clean is good, but if I can't sustain it, I need to try something new."

Your Turn

1. Your partner keeps asking you for large amounts of money. You feel uncomfortable but you're afraid of being abandoned. You think, "Just once more is okay." *What can you ask yourself to see it in a new way?*

    Question: I would ask myself, "_____?"
    Answer: I would answer by saying, "_____

    _____

    _____

    _____."

2. You're having horrible memories of being assaulted. The pictures keep replaying in your mind and you can't shut them off. You think, "I can't live this way. I want to die." *What can you ask yourself to see it in a new way?*

    Question: I would ask myself, "_____?"
    Answer: I would answer by saying, "_____

    _____

    _____

    _____."

3. You have a toothache that's getting worse. You try to ignore it. You're in a lot of pain, but you hate going to the dentist. You keep putting it off. *What can you ask yourself to see it in a new way?*

    Question: I would ask myself, "_____?"
    Answer: I would answer by saying, "_____

_____

_____

_____."

4. You've been putting up a good front. No one knows you're struggling with addiction. But inside you're dying. You think, "I can't stop." *What can you ask yourself to see it in a new way?*

    Question: I would ask myself, "_____?"
    Answer: I would answer by saying, "_____

_____

_____

_____."

5. One of your situations: _____

_____

What can you ask yourself to see it in a new way?

    Question: I would ask myself, "_____?"
    Answer: I would answer by saying, "_____

_____

_____

_____."

Growth Exercise: *Create an Ideal to Live For*

It's essential to have some ideal that your life stands for. An ideal is any worthy cause that moves you, such as:

✦ "I want to improve the environment. We're destroying the planet, and while I'm here I want to do what I can to preserve nature."

✦ "I want to raise my children to be good people."

✦ "I want to paint. I feel most alive when I'm painting. Beauty can lift people up."

✦ "I want to help kids who were hurt like I was. I want them to know it's not their fault, and that someone is there for them."

✦ "I want to devote my life to my religion. I believe religion can create peace in the world."

Ideals are outside the self. They contribute to progress in the world. What are not ideals? Any goals that are limited to just the physical realm or just to yourself. For example, making money is necessary for everyone, but it's not an ideal. If you expand it to, "I want to make money so I can travel and learn," or, "I want to make money so I can give my children an education," these are now ideals. The money is not the goal, but it's a way to achieve something larger.

Because ideals are always invisible, it's easy to lose sight of their importance, to think they don't really exist or don't matter. But if you talk to people who are living a life of fulfillment or genuine achievement (not just work success), you'll find they have some ideal they care about. An ideal is like a compass or star that guides you. It helps you decide what's worth spending time on, what to do with your day.

Now think of addiction: there is no ideal in it. Using a substance may have been fun or pleasurable, but it's not leading anywhere. It's just for the moment; it does not last. Indeed, one study of addicted women found they used substances to "find a degree of . . . purpose otherwise missing from their lives" (Taylor 1998, 77). Substances never bring that in the long run because they don't serve a larger vision.

Imagine you are elderly, looking back: what will you want your life to have been about? We all leave a legacy. What will yours be? Remember that continuing your addiction is a legacy, too: one of hurting yourself and others through wasted talent and opportunity. Even if you grew up in a family where there were no ideals, you can create one now. Everyone needs something to live for. The poet Langston Hughes said, "When dreams die, life is a broken-winged bird that cannot fly" (Hughes 1994). The paradox is that when you devote yourself to a cause outside yourself, you become your truest self.

The ideal you choose does not have to be a career. You may be lucky and find gratifying work. Or you may have a job that just pays the bills. But you can always move toward your ideal, perhaps by going back to school, taking a class or volunteering a few hours a week. The key is not to wait. Ideals need to be brought alive, like a flame.

Some people come up with a reason they can't start now. You may think you need to get clean first, for example. But by making even small steps toward your ideal, you're making recovery more likely. As you give up addiction, replacing it with meaningful activity gives you a reason to go on. You may think you're too busy already and can't possibly add one more thing. This goes back to the basic question: what are you busy at, if not some larger purpose in life?

How?

Identify here any ideals that appeal to you; add your own as well. Where it says "list here," fill in what specifically you want to do.

Ideal	Not at all appealing	A little appealing	Moderately appealing	Extremely appealing
Creativity (e.g., painting, music, writing, dance) List here: _____ _____	0	1	2	3
Helping people (e.g., the poor, elderly, women, children) List here: _____ _____	0	1	2	3
Advocacy (e.g., the environment, politics, a charity) List here: _____ _____	0	1	2	3
Spirituality (e.g., a religion, meditation) List here: _____ _____	0	1	2	3
Your family (e.g., raising your children well) List here: _____ _____	0	1	2	3
Other: _____ _____ List here: _____ _____	0	1	2	3

Now go back and circle at least one ideal you can commit to now, even in a small way. It may be the one highest on the list, or the one that is most realistic for your life these days.

Write about your ideal. Why is it important? What will it bring you?

_____

_____

_____

_____

_____

_____

_____

Find a way to make this ideal more present in your life. Check off any approach that you want to use:

✦ Volunteer a few hours a week. (You can ask a librarian how to locate volunteer opportunities, call the United Way, or look in the Yellow Pages.)

✦ Locate others who are making this type of effort (e.g., by contacting a charity or church).

✦ Read, search the Internet, or take a class to find out more.

✦ Other: _____

Growth Exercise: *Rethink*

Rethinking means "talking yourself through" a difficult situation. Do you ever notice that all through the day, you're having a conversation with yourself? Everyone does this. It's not like the "talking to yourself" that means you're mentally ill. This internal voice that we all have is also called *self-talk*.

If you grew up in a home that was nurturing, you would have learned a nurturing voice. The supportive voice of your parents would have become your own internal voice. Unfortunately, many people grew up hearing a harsh voice. They learned to yell at themselves. And others have a mixed voice—at times nurturing, at times harsh.

Women with addiction often have a very harsh voice. They beat themselves up for just about everything. As Kasl (1992) has noted, men with addiction often have an inflated ego and need humility; AA was founded on this principle. In contrast, many women and minorities already have a "crushed, nonexistent ego" and they need to have "their egos built up through celebration, validation" (Kasl 1992, 19).

You may believe that it's right to have a harsh voice, that you deserve it: "I screwed up and am just being accurate." You may think that a harsh voice will lead you to change your addictive behavior, but the opposite is true. A nurturing voice leads to growth. This does not mean you're being easy on yourself or telling yourself everything you do is fine. It's a voice of accountability and truth, but with kindness. A major task in recovery is developing that supportive voice. This is not a voice that comes naturally; usually your automatic thoughts are harsh and blaming. Rethinking means being supportive and truthful at the same time.

How?

The first step is to create an image of a supportive voice. After that, you can try using that supportive voice to rethink one of your difficult life situations.

Step I: Create an Image

It may help to develop an image of your nurturing voice. The image can be one of those offered below or any other that you choose. At first it may be easier to tap into a supportive voice through imagining what someone else might say. As you practice, that voice can become your own. Circle any that you like, or write about your own image.

+ **A good coach or manager**. When you think of a good sports coach or manager at work, how does that person talk? She tries to motivate you to do your best. The good coach knows your strengths and weaknesses and seeks to help you improve. The good coach might say, "Stay focused—stick to it and you'll get there."

+ **A loving parent**. If you had a loving parent, you can draw on that experience. Even if you didn't, you have an idea of what a loving parent sounds like. You can think of a loving parent you saw on TV or in the movies. You can make this voice a mix of the people who represent this style, such as a caring teacher, therapist, or priest. The loving parent guides you through tough times. The loving parent might say, "You have a lot to offer. You can get through this. We can work on the problem."

+ **Someone who talks you down**. Think of the 6 o'clock news, with the story of a person about to jump off a building. There's always someone there trying to talk the person down. That person says supportively: "You have a lot to live for," or, "Whatever's bothering you can get worked out." You can learn to "talk yourself down" from the emotional ledge you're on at times.

Your image of a supportive voice:

_____

_____

_____

_____

_____

_____

_____

Step II: Rethink

Here's an in-depth example of rethinking. Then, you can try it out using a situation from your own life.

Example

Carol's *situation*: Carol is lonely. She thought that by now she'd be in a long-term relationship. Instead, she's alone with a string of failed relationships behind her.

Carol's *thinking*: "You're such a loser. No one wants you. You're never going to find anyone."

This is the first voice that pops into Carol's mind. It's her automatic voice. She could go on and on like this, being mean to herself. This voice is harsh. It only talks in a negative way. It's not balanced or fair. It does not lead to growth.

Carol's *rethinking*: "It's true you're alone. You expected life to be different. But it doesn't mean you have to get depressed or drink. You can learn to build a lasting relationship. Maybe you could work on how to pick the right person and how to deal with conflicts. No one taught you these skills when you were young because yours was such a messed up family; no one ever talked about anything real. You can learn now. You can read about relationships, take a class, talk to people, go to therapy, get out more to meet people. You can develop yourself so you feel more attractive and confident. There's a lot you can do to turn the situation around. You're a human being like everyone else, and that means you can develop a relationship if you have enough guidance and support, and if you do what it takes. You're a good person and you just need to work on this area of your life."

This is the voice that Carol has to work to get to. It doesn't come automatically—she has to sit and rethink to tap into it. The voice takes effort but leads to growth. It's supportive but realistic. It seeks to solve the problem rather than just blame. It feels hopeful but truthful too.

How *Not* to Rethink

Let's also look at how not to rethink. People often believe that rethinking means positive thinking, as in the phrase, "Don't worry, be happy!" or the character Stuart Smalley on the TV show *Saturday Night Live* who said, "I'm good enough, I'm smart enough, and doggone it, people like me." But this isn't it. Rethinking is *realistic, truthful thinking*. It's about looking at a situation honestly and seeing it fully. That includes positive and negative truths—holding on to both sides of the picture.

How would it sound if Carol, in the example above, just did positive thinking? She might say to herself, "You'll be fine! You're a great person and people like you! You'll find a partner soon. Just focus on the positive and it'll work out."

Do you notice what's wrong with this? It doesn't sound *real*. If you take negative thoughts and try to just make them positive, it doesn't work. Rethinking needs to be balanced.

Your Turn

Now try rethinking one of your life situations. You can model it on the example above. Make it sound like the image of the supportive voice you created earlier.

Your *situation*:

_____

_____

_____

_____

Your *thinking*:

_____

_____

_____

_____

Your *rethinking*:

_____

_____

_____

_____

Self-Awareness Summary

You can use this as a guide to remember the skills you want to keep learning.

How much do you *currently* use these coping skills?

	Not at all	A little helpful	Moderately	Extremely
Listen to that small, quiet voice	0	1	2	3
Ask questions	0	1	2	3
Create an ideal to live for	0	1	2	3
Rethink	0	1	2	3

How helpful would it be to use these coping skills *more*?

	Not at all helpful	A little helpful	Moderately helpful	Extremely helpful
Listen to that small, quiet voice	0	1	2	3
Ask questions	0	1	2	3
Create an ideal to live for	0	1	2	3
Rethink	0	1	2	3

CHAPTER 8

Healing Through Action

Action is the bottom line. It's a coded message, telling you how you're doing. There is often a gap between people's actions and their words. One can be smooth with words, but action can't be faked—it's either there or it's not.

With action, you watch yourself as if you're watching a movie. You see yourself eat a healthy meal and you think, "I must be okay; I'm taking care of my body." You see yourself saying "yes" to a drink on an airplane and think, "This isn't good—I told myself I wouldn't do this." Called an *observing ego*, part of you is watching what the rest of you is doing. It's a strength. It helps you choose a different action if your current behavior is unhealthy. If you're *impulsive*—acting without this observing ego—your actions are driving you, like the cart before the horse.

This chapter offers four growth exercises:

❈ Control an impulse

❈ Extreme self-care

❈ Do one thing you're afraid of every day

❈ Take charge

It might be said that we are what we do. Actions define us. When you choose actions that are in line with your long-term goals and values, you feel good. As Abraham Lincoln said, "When I do good, I feel good. When I do bad, I feel bad. That's my religion." It's a simple, stark truth. When you live by it, life can become a waking dream. When you ignore it by pretending or wishing your actions don't matter, life can become a nightmare. The glory is that every day you have a new chance to start over. No matter what came before, you can choose *now* as the time to act in ways consistent with your best self. It truly never is too late.

❈ ═══ ❈

Growth Exercise: *Control an Impulse*

The nature of addiction is loss of control. You can't stop using and the substance owns you—it runs your life. A key skill is regaining control. When you learn to control your impulses, you build real personal power. It's now you who decides your actions. You take back your life.

Many impulses need to be controlled in addition to substance use. Binging on food, rage attacks, overspending, reckless driving, and physically hurting yourself, for example, are all impulse problems. They have in common an out-of-control feeling in the moment and deep regret afterward. All impulsive actions weaken you; they harm you and your relationships. They are like the eruption of a volcano, spreading chaos and destruction.

Part of why it's so hard to control an impulse is that it feels so very right in the moment. At the time of the impulse, your vision narrows. You believe you must do it. Your mind goes almost blank; you forget everything else you know (such as the consequences of your actions). It may even feel intensely pleasurable. Perhaps you get rage attacks and yell at your partner. Do you notice that the yelling may feel good? That release makes you feel powerful? It may feel like a "high," aside from the effect of any substance. Later you see how wrong the action was and vow never to repeat it. But then the cycle does repeat. All impulses have this pattern: intense urge, quick action that feels right, and later regret. Controlling the impulse feels all wrong, like you're depriving yourself.

Yet containing an impulse is more than just "having to be good" or "not getting what I want." Your impulses contain important information about what's going on inside you. Once you bring the impulse down, you can explore what triggered it. For example, if you control the impulse to yell at your partner, a lot of thoughts and feelings may come up. You may think that if you don't yell, your partner won't listen or do what you want. This may remind you of how, growing up, you were the youngest and never got your way. You may feel anxious about feeling weak yet again. You may believe you'll never get your needs met. You may feel lonely. This process is called *from action into words*—when you control your destructive action, you can learn to express in words what the underlying pain was about. This is essential for really getting to the bottom of the impulse and working it through. Impulsive action perpetuates the pain; controlling it and facing the feelings heals the pain. As the psychologist Kurt Lewin (1951, 86) said, "If you want to understand something, try changing it."

So how do you control impulses? You create an *impulse control plan* (ICP)—a sort of emergency response system that can be used anytime, anywhere, as soon as there are signs of danger. An ICP is a set of steps that serve as a buffer between you and the impulse. It creates a twenty-minute (or longer) delay so you won't act impulsively. It's a simple but effective method. It's a "time-out."

There are three key points to know about using an impulse control plan (ICP).

1. **It takes at least 15–20 minutes to bring your impulse down.** This is biologically wired; that's simply how long it takes for your brain and body to settle down after this animal-like urge.

2. **It helps to create an image to guide you.** For example, you might imagine pulling the reins on a horse that's bucking. Having a clear image can help, because in the midst of an impulse your ability to think is limited. Returning to the same image over and over is a shortcut.

3. **In the long run, you'll need to explore the feelings underlying the impulse.** All impulses are signs of important feelings that need to be explored. An ICP will bring the impulse down. It's a "first aid" response. Later you'll need to deal with the underlying injury and pain.

How?

Create your own impulse control plan using the three steps here.

Step I: Create an Image

The image you create can be anything to remind you to control the impulse. Some are listed below, or you can create your own. Really picture it in your mind, using your senses to hear it, see it, smell it, and touch it. You can also draw the image or find a photo or other symbolic object; for example, a citation for driving while under the influence or a photo of your child (anything that reminds you of the consequences of your impulse).

☐ Pulling the reins on a horse that's bucking.

☐ Pulling the leash on a dog that's running away.

☐ S-l-o-w-i-n-g d-o-w-n, like a slow motion movie.

☐ Shutting an iron gate—you turn your back on all the destruction behind you.

☐ Other: _____

Step II: Name the Activities in Your Impulse Control Plan

Choose whatever activities will distract you from the impulse. It needs to take at least twenty minutes. Check off as many as you like, or think of your own. It may work best to always do the same activities in the same order. Or you can use different ones at different times, depending on time of day and where you are.

☐ Take a shower, making the water either as warm or cold as possible.

☐ Take a walk outside.

☐ Listen to calming music.

☐ Sing.

☐ Exercise.

☐ Read.

☐ Do a hobby or craft.

☐ Call someone.

☐ Watch TV.

☐ Eat a meal slowly.

☐ Meditate.

☐ Clean your house.

☐ Play a game.

☐ Work on a task, such as paying bills.

☐ Drink a cup of tea.

☐ Write in your journal.

☐ Other: _____

☐ Other: _____

Step III: Rate How You're Feeling

After the twenty minutes of your ICP, rate whether your impulse has gone down enough that you no longer feel in danger of acting impulsively.

0	1	2	3
Not at all impulsive	A little impulsive	Moderately impulsive	Extremely impulsive

If you rated 0, you're fine. If you rated 1, 2, or 3, do another twenty minutes of your ICP. People often have to repeat the ICP several times—that's fine; just keep going until you're back to safety.

Growth Exercise: *Extreme Self-Care*

Extreme self-care is like *extreme sports*—it means going to the ultimate. It's the idea that you need to do more than just the basics in taking care of yourself. You need to take it on as a mission, a huge priority, as front-and-center of your life.

The world has speeded up and there's enormous pressure on many people. Women especially are balancing more roles than ever before. They often have primary responsibility for children while working outside the home. They may be taking care of elderly parents, who are now living longer. If you are like most women, you feel deluged keeping up with family, work, money, chores, social life, eating right, working out, keeping up your appearance, and—when you can find the time—leisure. In fact, the number one stress that most women report is a lack of time. Women working full-time with children under the age of thirteen are the most stressed group of all (McKenna 1998).

In earlier times people stayed put and were tied to extended family and community. Now you may have the disorientation of starting anew several times during your life and having to build bonds in each place. It's widely noted that there's less community support and more isolation than in previous eras (Putnam 2000). All this adds up to feeling more alone while at the same time having to do more.

Thus, you need to take good care of yourself. Women, however, often take care of everyone else, leaving themselves for last. Addiction adds to this pattern, as it always involves some degree of poor self-care. In addiction, you are saying your body doesn't matter, your peace of mind doesn't matter—what matters is using the substance. Indeed, Covington defines addiction as "a chronic neglect of self in favor of something or someone else" (2000, 16). If you grew up around people with addiction or were neglected as a child, your problems in self-care may go back a long way.

In this growth exercise, the goal is to counter these trends—make self-care your top priority. Everything flows from that. You'll take better care of others if you're taking care of yourself. You'll more likely stay clean and sober because you're fulfilling your needs. Indeed, just getting seven to eight hours of sleep a night and eating breakfast are associated with less substance use (Sanders-Phillips 1998). You'll like yourself more, because you're living a life of self-respect.

How?

Draw a *heart* next to each item below that you will do to improve your self-care. Put a *star* next to those you are already doing (good for you!). Also, you can change any item to fit you better (e.g., number of times per week). You don't have to do them all, but the goal is to move beyond your current level of self-care. Make it realistic, but aim high!

_____ Have at least one hour a day just for you.

_____ Take a walk every day.

_____ Drink 6 to 8 glasses of water per day.

_____ Eat healthier food _____ (lower fat? more vegetables? less junk food?).

_____ Take vitamins daily.

_____ Do at least 20 minutes of exercise 3 times per week.

_____ Spend _____ minutes a day to keep your car/office/home free of clutter.

_____ Do one fun social event each week.

_____ Get annual medical, dental, eye, and gynecologic exams.

_____ Read something you enjoy at least _____ minutes a day.

_____ Write in your journal every day.

_____ Get a massage once every _____ (week? month?).

_____ Take a day-trip or weekend away every _____ (month? season?).

_____ Go to a cultural event that inspires you every _____ (week? month? season?).

_____ Do a spiritual practice (e.g., church, temple, meditation) every _____ (day? week?).

_____ Practice safe sex.

_____ Engage in a creative activity (e.g. drawing, painting, dance) every _____ (day? week?).

_____ Get enough sleep.

_____ Do recovery activities (e.g., treatment, AA) every _____ (day? week?).

_____ Have a date with your partner each _____ (week? month?).

_____ Other: _____

_____ Other: _____

Yes, But . . .

Now it's time to counter the "yes, but. . ." thoughts that are likely coming up. Put a check next to any thoughts you notice:

____ I don't have time.

____ It costs too much.

____ It won't make a difference.

____ I don't matter enough.

____ Other people are more important.

____ I can't get myself to do it.

____ Other: _____

How to respond to these? Dig down deep. These thoughts that pop up are surface thoughts. There's a deeper side of you that is wiser and smarter, that can see through these excuses. For example, if you say, "I don't have time," a response might sound like this:

"It's true that you're busy. But why are you always choosing other priorities? Why are you so willing to devote time to just about anything but yourself? You give time to work, family, church—pretty much everywhere else. That's not fair. In the long run you're wearing yourself down. You feel tired and you're drinking too much—can you see what's happening? I know it's scary and unfamiliar to put yourself first, but you need to. Try it and see what happens. You know the old ways aren't working."

Extreme self-care asks you to go to an extreme—to really, truly make it happen no matter what. There will be many "yes, but . . ." thoughts that arise as you try to do it. You may start out strong, then go back to your old pattern. Figure out what you need to do to make this practice airtight; to make it a promise, on your word, that you'll stick to. Extreme solutions are required for extreme self-care!

Write down below what efforts you'll make for extreme self-care to become a reality rather than just another good idea that falls by the wayside. You might copy this page to post on your refrigerator so you'll see it every day. You could schedule times for self-care activities in your daily calendar. You could find a friend to do it with, and remind each other. You can also think up other ways to make it happen.

_____

_____

_____

Growth Exercise:
Do One Thing You're Afraid of Every Day

This is a simple, but profound idea: Do one thing you fear every day. It might be saying something you're afraid to say, sitting down to pay the bills, writing, returning an item to a store, or cleaning your house. Do you feel the energy drain that comes when these are hanging over you? They weigh on you. They sap you. They create tension. As Eleanor Roosevelt said, "You must do the thing which you think you cannot do."

It feels like taking a leap off the high dive: you jump with your heart in your throat. For most people, it doesn't feel good to start—you feel you're doing it all wrong, you'll never get it done, you're not good enough. But you get in a groove, you "flow," and the thing happens. These same feelings happen whether you're doing something simple like cleaning your car or something complex like writing a paper for school.

Why do one thing every day? It's like an athletic workout. It builds endurance. What you are really creating is self-discipline, which is the driving force behind much in life. It heals addiction, because addiction is about letting go of responsibility, about giving in. If you do at least one thing every day, you'll find it becomes a habit. As addiction is a bad habit, doing what you fear is a good habit.

Over time, you can do more and more. You'll feel good about what you're accomplishing. Indeed, it's one of the best ways to build self-esteem. People sometimes think self-esteem comes just from saying nice things to yourself, but far more powerful is seeing yourself do what you know you need to do.

The key is just to do it every day like clockwork. That keeps the momentum going. It's been said that "If you leave it for a day, it will leave you for two." It's harder to jump back in once you procrastinate.

This skill may be especially important for women, because traditionally they are not raised to overcome their fears as much as men. Boys are socialized to be strong, to do tough things (perhaps too much), while girls may not be as encouraged to do what is hard. Thus, this skill is also about learning independence and self-reliance.

Even if you are successful in many parts of your life, you have fears—everyone does. Such fears may be around showing vulnerability—letting people know how much you hurt or that you need help. These are common fears in people who are highly competent.

You may think you need to feel motivated first and then you'll do what you're afraid of. But you'll find it's the opposite—if you take the leap, you'll develop more motivation over time. Success breeds success.

Finally, notice your patterns. Some people prefer getting it over first thing in the morning; others wait until they're geared up, late in the day. Like getting into a pool, some dip a toe in the water while others jump right in. Either way is fine, as long as you end up swimming! Similarly, some people start with the hardest items on their list while others begin with the easiest and move up. There's no right or wrong, as long as you make it happen.

Here are some tips to help you take the leap:

+ **Try it for just ten minutes.** It can feel less scary if you know it's just for ten minutes, and then you can quit. Often you'll find that after ten minutes, you're in the groove and want to keep going.

+ **You "win" no matter how it turns out.** You get credit for making the effort. If it goes well, great. If not, you can still learn from it.

+ **Use self-soothing.** Talk yourself through it very gently. See the growth exercise Soothe Yourself in chapter 9.

+ **Do it, no matter how you feel.** It's normal to feel overwhelmed, hopeless, unsure, worried. That's okay—it will get easier, guaranteed.

+ **Do something, anything.** You don't have to do it wonderfully or pick the best approach. Just start anywhere.

How?

Now, it's time to think about what you fear, and to try a simple experiment of facing that fear. Good luck!

Step 1: Make a List

What are you afraid of doing? Write a list below, including everything from day-to-day basics to the big goals of your life. Be sure they're specific, such as "Sign up for a course at the community college this semester" or "Ask my mother to stop criticizing how I raise the kids." List them from "least afraid" (on line 1) to "most afraid" (on line 10). Don't worry if they're not ranked perfectly—just try to get a general sense.

1. _____ **(Least afraid)**

2. _____

3. _____

4. _____

5. _____

6. _____

7. _____

8. _____

9. _____

10. _____ **(Most afraid)**

Step II: Predict, Then Find Out

Usually people fear doing something because they imagine something bad will happen. It can help to compare your prediction to reality. Take one item from your list and fill in the following chart. Fill out the "before" section now, and the "after" section once you've done that item. An example is provided. Photocopy this page and the next page for each of the items on your list, if you want.

Example

Item __8__ from my list: *"Tell my mother not to criticize how I raise the kids."*

Before

What I'm afraid will happen:

I think she'll hate me. She'll say I'm not a good mother. I'll be hurt and guilty.

After

What actually happened

I told her it bothers me when she keeps telling me how to raise the children. She said that she just cares about them a lot. She said she'd try not to keep doing it. She seemed a little upset, but didn't say anything mean. I'm glad I finally said it.

Your Turn

Now you try it.

Item _____ from my list:

Before

What I'm afraid will happen:

_____

_____

_____

_____

After

What actually happened:

_____

_____

_____

_____

Step III: Notice Your Reactions

What insights did you gain? For example, how difficult was it to do the thing you feared? Do you feel relieved? What would you do differently next time? How do you feel about yourself now? What did you learn?

_____

_____

_____

_____

_____

_____

Growth Exercise: *Take Charge*

"Taking charge" means you are captain of your ship. If recovery is a voyage, you are the leader—you make the decisions, you protect yourself from danger, and you solve problems that arise. Whether skies are sunny or stormy, you find a way to move forward.

Everyone who succeeds in recovery will tell you the same thing: "At some point, I decided it was up to me." This doesn't mean they did it alone. They will tell you that they relied on others' wisdom and advice. But ultimately they understood that "the buck stops here." In the words of Women for Sobriety, "I am responsible for myself and my actions."

This can be both freeing and frightening. It's freeing because you recognize that you have the power to steer your life in the direction you want it to go. It's frightening because it means no one can save you from yourself. You must become your own advocate, best friend, problem solver, and coach. Once you get used to it, however, you won't want to go back. People who acquire power never willingly give it up.

What does taking charge look like day to day? It means you continually look for opportunities to do the "right thing"—recovery activities, building relationships with safe people, being productive, and getting rest when you need it. It means you work on the life problems you identified in chapters 3 and 4 of this book (and any others you are aware of). It means you develop your talents. It means you ask for feedback about how you're doing. It means you take a "lockdown" approach to protecting yourself from danger: you set firm boundaries. It means when you hit rough spots you actively seek solutions rather than passively sitting back, wishing and fantasizing that things will work out or that someone will bail you out. You say to yourself, "What's the best action I can take right now to make my life go better?" This becomes your mantra, your filter through which every decision is made. You view time as your major resource in life. You think in terms of *now* rather than *tomorrow*.

Women often give up their power too easily. They may stay in relationships where they're being used by others. At work, they may become primarily the helpers of men rather than focusing on their own career needs. They may be overly concerned with appearance or fitting in. They may come to value being liked more than liking themselves. When women do these things, it's often unconscious—they're not aware they've handed their personal power over to others. Growing up, they may have absorbed subtle messages about "women's place." It's not that women should give up being a helper to others—it's a great strength to nurture and caretake. But when helping becomes so extreme that you lose yourself, it's time to change.

Taking charge also means accurately seeing how you became addicted. You seek to find out the truth, even if it's painful. You take a balanced view, understanding the wide array of forces behind addiction—family history, biology, emotional problems, life issues, cultural influences. But you also see that it was you who chose to keep picking up the substance rather than stopping when it became too much. You own your part, while also seeing the complexity of addiction.

If addiction was in your family when you were growing up, you may have had poor models of how to take charge. You may have learned unhealthy lessons: give in to a substance when times get tough; escape pain with drugs; pretend addiction is okay. If you absorbed such messages as a child, it will be even more important to counter these with a take-charge approach now.

In relationships, a take-charge approach means that even if no one around you supports your recovery, you support it. You recognize that you have every right to feel disappointed if your partner, parents, and family are not supportive. But you don't let this get in the way of reaching out to find people who *can* be there for you.

A wonderful paradox occurs if you are willing to accept this role that life gives you. The more you take charge, the more good things seem to come out of nowhere—opportunities land in your lap, people appear. The paradox is that when you take control, random good luck seems to increase as well.

As children, we looked to parents to take charge, but now it's up to us. You can still have childlike sides, but the adult side needs to grow too.

How?

Answer the questions here to see how much you take charge of your life. After that, you can decide what next steps are right for you.

Step 1: Explore

Answer each of the following questions. Be honest. If you're not sure about some, ask others who know you well for feedback.

1. When one thing doesn't work, I almost always look for another solution (rather than giving up).	Yes	No
2. I have a circle of people I can call on for advice about my recovery (e.g., sponsor, therapist, doctor, clean and sober friends).	Yes	No
3. I can say "no" to unhealthy or excessive demands from others.	Yes	No
4. If I want to use a substance, I almost always do something to prevent it rather than giving in (e.g., call someone, delay, rethink, go to a meeting, distract myself).	Yes	No
5. I make the major decisions in my life, even if I get input from others.	Yes	No
6. I do not allow people to abuse me (e.g., physically, sexually, verbally, financially).	Yes	No
7. I believe in taking charge of my life, rather than hoping someone else will fix it.	Yes	No
8. I spend at least thirty hours a week in productive activity (e.g., work, school, raising children, volunteering, recovery activities, treatment, housekeeping, hobbies, reading, exercise, chores).	Yes	No
9. I reach out for help when I'm overwhelmed or in danger.	Yes	No
10. I take action to solve the life problems I identified in chapters 3 and 4 of this book.	Yes	No
11. Recovery is my highest priority.	Yes	No
12. I take charge of my health care (e.g., choosing doctors, asking questions).	Yes	No

Step II: Create a Plan

How could you take charge more? Write your ideas here. You can draw from what you discovered in filling out the questionnaire. You can list how you want to take charge. You can explore the messages you got about taking charge when you were growing up. Write whatever you think will help you.

_____

_____

_____

_____

_____

_____

Self-Awareness Summary

You can use this guide to remember the skills you want to keep learning.

How much do you *currently* use these coping skills?

	Not at all	A little	Moderately	Extremely
Control an impulse	0	1	2	3
Extreme self-care	0	1	2	3
Do one thing you're afraid of every day	0	1	2	3
Take charge	0	1	2	3

How helpful would it be to use these coping skills *more*?

	Not at all helpful	A little helpful	Moderately helpful	Extremely helpful
Control an impulse	0	1	2	3
Extreme self-care	0	1	2	3
Do one thing you're afraid of every day	0	1	2	3
Take charge	0	1	2	3

CHAPTER 9

Healing Through Feelings

Feelings are both the most wonderful and the most awful experiences human beings have. You can feel joy, love, energy; you can feel despair, bitterness, hatred—and everything in between. Yet many people never learn, growing up, how to work with feelings. Feelings are sometimes not even discussed.

In this chapter the growth exercises are designed to help you become comfortable with your full range of feelings. You gain mastery, moving into feelings to experience them more fully and moving away from them when they are too intense. Feelings do not have to feel dangerous or out of control. They can become the source of a life fully lived.

The four growth exercises are:

- Soothe yourself
- Choose self-respect
- Mourn
- Accept

A key idea is that no feelings are bad; all are there for a reason. If you honor them, they will repay you. If you ignore them, they will haunt you. You may say, "I shouldn't feel angry" or "I shouldn't feel upset." You may feel weak, defective, or even monstrous for having certain feelings. But there are no "shoulds" with feelings—feelings simply *are*, and the goal is to let them guide you. Anger and upset are important clues, for example, that can help protect you if you are willing to hear their message.

Sometimes you may not be fully aware of your feelings. Becoming conscious is part of the work. You can bring feelings from underground into the light.

Women are sometimes criticized for being "too emotional." This stereotype can be harmful if it assumes that the goal is to be unemotional. Feelings, when understood, are a source of strength. Women may have a particular talent for intuition and connection, for example. Thus, the goal isn't to get rid of feelings, but to learn to modulate them.

Ultimately, dealing with feelings is about love. You say to yourself, "I'm not going to pretend the pain doesn't matter. I'm not going to neglect or punish you. I want to hear what you feel. You deserve to be heard." Isn't that how you would aim to treat someone you care about?

Feelings are the true high in life, more than substances.

Growth Exercise: *Soothe Yourself*

Addiction is often about trying to soothe yourself, but in ways that end up hurting you. People who don't understand addiction sometimes think that substances don't really make you feel better. But they can—alcohol can calm you and cocaine can give you energy, for example. Once you're addicted, you realize the cost is too high—the quick fix results in serious problems.

Thus, it's important to soothe yourself without a substance. Soothing means finding a way to feel better—by talking gently to yourself or doing a calming activity (taking a bath, watching a movie).

Soothing may sound childlike. Indeed, it's exactly what you do with a small child. But it's also something that everyone—including adults—needs at times. It comes naturally if you were reassured a lot as a child; you would now just do that with yourself. But if you weren't treated this way, you may not know how, or you may view it as "stupid" or "embarrassing." You should know that healthy adults soothe themselves often.

You may say, "But soothing doesn't work as well as a substance." Early in recovery, you may be right. Soothing is not as quick or powerful. But over time, you'll find that you won't miss the substance. Indeed, Fletcher (2001) found that 86 percent of people in recovery found they didn't miss their substance once they had been clean for a number of years. For now, soothing may seem like it can't compete with the substance, but later it will be more than enough.

Soothing is especially important as a way to bring down intense negative feelings. All destructive action occurs when you have a negative feeling that gets out of hand. It might be anger that bursts into a rage attack, a craving that turns into drinking, or anxiety that becomes a food binge. When you think of your own destructive actions, was there some intense negative feeling that led up to them?

The goal is therefore to bring down negative feelings when they reach the danger zone. People sometimes think they should always "get in touch with" or "express" their feelings. But when a negative feeling is overwhelming, you need to reduce it to a safe level. You contain the feeling. You control it rather than letting it control you. Later you can figure it out. What is the danger zone? Usually, it's when any negative feeling goes above 6 on a 0 to 10 scale, where 0 "means not at all" and 10 means "extremely". For example, if your anger level is at an eight, it's time to bring it down. Soothing is one of the best ways to do this.

Finally, note that some soothing activities can themselves become addictions (e.g., food, sex). You'll want to notice whether these are becoming addictive for you. But generally, as you give up a substance you may use such activities more for a while and it won't be a problem. You may gain weight or eat more sugar, for example. Later you can get back to normal.

How?

When you think of how to soothe a child, there are two main ways. One is to *talk* to the child in a very kind, reassuring way. The second is to get the child involved in a calming *activity*. These two ways work for adults as well—and healthy adults use them often! Read the example here. After that you can try practicing soothing.

Example

Example of talking to yourself in a soothing way: "You're a good person, you can get through this. It's okay to have feelings about this, but right now, just stay centered. Keep perspective. You can figure it out later. Get back to a good place—safe and calm. From there, you can do anything. Don't let this drag you down. You can solve the problem later. Take care of yourself for now."

Examples of soothing activities:

✦ Play with a pet or child

✦ Eat a favorite food

✦ Get something done (e.g., laundry)

✦ Take a walk in the sun

✦ Watch a movie

✦ Take a bath

✦ Listen to music

✦ Call a friend

✦ Read

✦ Do artwork

✦ Your favorite soothing activities? _____

_____

Example of a real-life situation

"It's 8 P.M. I just got home from work and I'm beat. I want a drink to relax."

How could you soothe yourself without a drink?

"I would tell myself that I need to do something nice, but it can't be a drink. I might have a hot soak in the tub. I might call my friend Paula and chat for a while. I guess I could eat something or get a cappuccino. I would say to myself, 'You deserve better than a drink. A drink will make you feel bad later. Treat yourself well.'"

Your Turn

Write out how you could soothe yourself through each situation.

1. "I want to call up my ex-boyfriend. I know he really hurt me, but I miss him."
   How could you soothe yourself without calling someone you know is bad for you?

_____

_____

_____

2. "I weighed myself and I'm too fat. I want to go back to diet pills. They kept me thin."
   How could you soothe yourself without pills?

_____

_____

_____

3. "I've had a bad day and am about to explode. I want to scream because my partner forgot to take out the garbage."
   How could you soothe yourself without screaming at someone?

_____

_____

_____

4. "I spent my last paycheck on cocaine. I have almost no money. I want to get high and forget about all this."
   How could you soothe yourself without getting high?

_____

_____

_____

How About Your Life?

Now take situations from your own life where you think soothing could help. Write out how you would do it, as in the practice situations above. Choose situations that are truly difficult for you. Really work this!

1. _____

   How could you soothe yourself?

_____

_____

_____

2. _____

How could you soothe yourself?

_____

_____

_____

_____

3. _____

How could you soothe yourself?

_____

_____

_____

_____

Growth Exercise: *Choose Self-Respect*

Self-respect is a feeling. It says "I matter." It's defiant and proud. When you have this feeling, life can throw you curveballs, but you dodge them. Job stress, divorce, racism—whatever happens, you say "I'm not going to let this drag me down. I'm not going to use over it." It's a feeling of persistence and inner core. It says "I know hardships happen, but I can be like a tree solidly planted in the ground." It's a wise elder. It's a strong heart.

Self-respect tells you how to be and it also tells you how not to be. It says it's not okay to wake up drunk and miss work. It's not okay to let someone treat you badly. It not okay to drive high and endanger people around you.

If you tap into this feeling, you say "yes" to life. You say, "I'm going to make the best of the cards I've been dealt. I'm going to do what it takes. I don't want to leave this world with cirrhosis, overdosing, dying in a car wreck, or leaving my kids to fend for themselves." In the end, this is all we really have—to say, "My life matters." From this feeling, all else follows. You know what choices to make. You relate better to yourself and other people. You think differently. The confusion and agonizing fall away.

It's said that in life you have four glass balls: your health, your relationships, your work, and your integrity. You're juggling these four balls and if you drop one, it shatters. You want to hold them carefully.

With addiction, you may be so used to disliking yourself that you forget what it's like not to feel this way—not to go through the day pretending, not to live the lie, not to have two voices competing in your head, not to wake up ashamed of what you did last night. If you grew up under difficult circumstances you may not have learned to respect yourself. Thus, it's all the more important to create self-respect now, to move beyond the limited vision that was given to you.

How?

In this growth exercise, you're asked to imagine the feeling of self-respect, and then look at how you would be different if you chose to live by it.

Step 1: Tap into the Feeling

The first step is to get in touch with the feeling of self-respect. It's like noticing the difference between tension versus relaxation; it's an entirely different state. Once you know it, you can keep coming back to it. Try any of the following.

✦ **Find a role model.** Sometimes it's easiest to see self-respect in others. Observe someone who has it. How does she carry herself? How do people talk to her? What's the impression she leaves? How do you feel after you've spent time with her?

✦ **Create a symbol.** Bring self-respect alive; make it real. Just because it's invisible doesn't mean it's not there. You can carry something in your pocket that reminds you of it (e.g., your AA token, a copy of your child's birth certificate, a poem, or a quotation). Or you can remember a time when you felt self-respect and find a symbol for that (e.g., a photo of you at a younger age, or at a graduation).

✦ **Do a word painting.** With a word painting, you take the words below in any order you want and you add to them, writing for as long as you want. You let them take you wherever they're going to go. Like playing with paint on a canvas, you get loose. It doesn't have to be logical; it's about getting to feelings. You can use just some of the words or all of them:

  ✦ Self-respect
  ✦ Value
  ✦ Strong
  ✦ Weak
  ✦ Careful
  ✦ Love
  ✦ When?

  + Work

  + Time

  + Addiction

  + Hate

  + Wake up

  ✦ **Say it.** Find a way to say it to yourself. For example: "I won't let myself be treated badly. I belong on this earth as much as anyone. I get only one body and I will take care of it."

Use the space below to explore self-respect in any of the ways described above or any other you prefer.

_____

_____

_____

_____

_____

_____

_____

_____

_____

_____

Step II: Notice What Would Be Different

Now, explore how your life would be different if it drew more from a stance of self-respect. How would day-to-day life be different? Would you say goodbye to some relationships? How would you handle money? Would you work more or less? Would your addiction change? How would you care for your body? Would you dress differently? What kind of parent would you be? Fill in the blanks, writing what you know deep down that you need to write.

Example: If I chose self-respect, I would _make time to work out at the health club at least three times a week._

If I chose self-respect, I would _____

_____

If I chose self-respect, I would _____

_____

If I chose self-respect, I would _____

_____

If I chose self-respect, I would _____

_____

If I chose self-respect, I would _____

_____

If I chose self-respect, I would _____

_____

Growth Exercise: *Mourn*

Grieving is part of life. Everyone faces disappointments, losses, and death. When these happen, it's important to let yourself have the feelings that arise—the sadness, anger, upset. Unfortunately, many people become blocked and do not go through the normal grief process. Growing up, they may have learned they shouldn't cry, or may have seen family members ignore feelings rather than working them through. Some people may have had too many painful experiences; they're afraid if they start to cry they'll never stop.

Many women with addiction have unresolved grief. It's common to reach for a substance as a way to kill the pain of loss—the loss of trust from child abuse, the loss of a partner (through breakup or divorce), the loss of youth with aging, the death of someone close. Substance abuse itself creates great losses as well: wasted years, opportunities, and relationships. Giving up a substance, too, is described as loss, like a best friend or lover now gone (Knapp 1997).

If you have unresolved grief, you may not know how to mourn. You may believe it's better to just move on rather than to fully feel a loss. You may believe grieving is the same as depression and should be avoided at all costs. You may believe you can't cry, or that you should be over what happened to you already. All of these are incorrect beliefs about grief, however.

Mourning is a process that can give you back to yourself—that can free you from the "ghosts" that haunt you. You can take it at your own pace, and eventually emerge on the other side.

How?

In this growth exercise, two steps are offered. The first is simply to learn more about grieving. The second offers actual mourning. It is very important that you carefully evaluate which steps you're ready for. The first (learning about grief) can be handled by anyone—it is only information. The second (actual mourning) should only be done if you're ready to handle it. When you get to that section, guidance is offered on how to decide. You'll see that it's strongly recommended that you seek professional help if you have major unresolved losses or are in danger of destructive action.

Step 1: Learning About Mourning

Key ideas on mourning are described here. As you read, put a check next to those that you understand and a question mark next to those you don't.

+ **Mourning and depression are different.** People often confuse them because they appear similar: both involve sadness and crying, for example. However they are different processes. Indeed, almost a hundred years ago Freud distinguished these in his famous essay "Mourning and Melancholia" (Freud 1917/1957).

  + *Mourning* is healthy and normal in response to loss. It has a beginning and end, and follows a natural course. After going through it, you feel resolved; you've worked through your grief. Indeed, every human culture has rituals and a time for mourning after a death because it's understood that mourning is an expected human process. The same process can be used for working through any loss.

  + *Depression* means you are stuck in sad feelings that you can't escape. It can go on for years, even a lifetime, if not treated. Ongoing depression is not a normal response to loss, and if it happens, you need professional help. (See chapter 4 for a description of depression.)

+ **It's a sign of strength to mourn.** Some people believe they should just be able to get over loss without having feelings. They think only "weak" people get upset. But it's normal to experience many feelings after a major loss, including grief, sadness, anger, hurt, and fear. Indeed, if you try to push them away, you're more likely to develop emotional problems such as depression, anxiety, addiction, or other issues. The phrase "the only way out is through" applies. This doesn't mean the mourning has to last a long time. You may find it brief or you may need a lot of time. And it's up to you to decide what counts as a real loss. One person may find divorce a major loss while another just feels relief. The key is to respect the feelings that arise and give yourself space and time to process them. Note too that no one can tell you that because your loss happened long ago, you should be over it already. If you were abused as a child, for example, it's common to mourn this only many years later. Also, if you've been addicted a long time, you may be able to mourn only once you've been clean from substances for a while.

✦ **Mourning is not just about crying.** Mourning does involve crying, but it's more than that. It's also about creating meaning—coming to terms with what happened and finding a reason to keep going on with your life. For example, if you lost someone very close or suffered child abuse, you may question whether life is good, whether you can ever love again, and why these losses exist. People find their own answers based on who they are and their spiritual beliefs. Mourning is thus about letting the feelings out, but also about resolving these larger meanings.

✦ **Mourning helps you grow as a person.** People often view mourning as "all bad," as purely pain. But successful mourning is one of the most profound emotional experiences people have. Yes, it's painful, but it also always gives back some gift—some positive new growth or understanding that you didn't have before. It might be a clearer sense of what matters to you in life. It might be a deeper sense of connection with others. It might be a positive shift in your career direction or relationships. You can't know in advance what those gifts will be, but just knowing that this happens can make it easier to go through the pain.

✦ **People often have mistaken views of crying.** For example, you may think that if you start to cry, you'll never stop. But this doesn't happen—the feelings always come back down. There's a natural beginning, middle, and end to each crying episode. You may have a number of episodes, but at the end of each, you'll stop. Human beings are simply not wired to cry forever. Think of how a child cries—it's intense, it comes back down, and then the child focuses on other things. Another belief about crying is, "I'm not able to cry." It's true that some people are blocked. You may need professional help to get you in touch with your feelings. But all people are capable of mourning if given guidance and support. Finally, some people believe that crying should be limited just to the immediate loss. But once the floodgates open, you may find pain from various past losses comes up. They may be all jumbled together and you feel it all at once. This is perfectly normal.

✦ **Readiness for mourning is essential.** You may say, "I'm ready to mourn now—I can handle it." Or you may think that you *should* be ready—you want to appear strong, even though you may not feel that way inside. It's essential to respect that mourning is a painful process and you must be truly prepared for it. It's dangerous to engage in mourning if you are currently acting in any destructive way toward yourself or others (e.g., physical harm or neglect, suicidal acts, or serious addiction). Bringing up feelings of loss when you don't yet have the coping skills to handle them can make you worse—you may use substances more or become suicidal. Also, if you have a history of many losses or childhood abuse, you will very likely need professional help to work through the pain. If you have depression or other emotional problems (see chapter 4), you should also seek professional help for mourning. Timing is important too: you may need to be in a solid place in your work life, housing, and supportive relationships. If you do not have these yet, you should likely wait. The key phrase is "When in doubt, don't"—if you have any reason to believe you're not ready for mourning, wait, get professional help, and pace it carefully. See the questions in the next section. Take care of yourself!

Step II: Actual Mourning

This section will describe actual ways of mourning. First, however, answer the following questions to help decide if you're ready. As discussed in the previous section, it's crucial to delay mourning until it's safe for you.

1. Do you currently have any self-destructive behavior (e.g., physical harm to self or others, serious addiction)?   Yes   No   Maybe

2. Do you believe you've had multiple severe losses (e.g., repeated child abuse, several deaths)?   Yes   No   Maybe

3. Do you believe it would be best to do mourning work with a professional? Yes   No   Maybe

4. In chapter 4, did you identify any current emotional problems? Yes   No   Maybe

5. Do you feel you're ready to face deep sadness?   Yes   No   Maybe

6. Do you want to do mourning now?   Yes   No   Maybe

Answers that indicate that you are ready to work on the rest of this section are: 1 = no; 2 = no; 3 = no; 4 = no; 5 = yes; 6 = yes. If you do not have this exact pattern, or if you have any "maybe" answers, please see a professional to help you decide and skip to the next growth exercise. Remember: stay safe in your recovery work. Never try to rush through or pretend you're further along than you are. Honor your experience.

Ways of Mourning

You can try any of the ways below to help you mourn. The idea is to let yourself just feel what comes up. Give yourself grieving space and time. You may also find the feelings come at odd moments when you don't expect them. Try to let yourself go through them whenever they arise (unless you are in a situation where that's impossible, such as a meeting at work). Respect what comes up, without pressure. It doesn't have to feel any particular way and you don't have to cry each time, for example. Become familiar with mourning—its ebb and flow. Notice too that you can choose when to move in and out of the feelings. You may also find that certain feelings turn into others as you do the work: anger may become sadness, for example. Please *be sure* to seek help if you notice any destructive behavior toward yourself or others, or if it becomes too overwhelming.

✦ Go to a place that reminds you of the loss. For example, go to a park where you spent time with a person who died.

✦ Look at photos that remind you.

✦ Join a grief support group. Even if your loss was not a death, you can often join such a group to work on whatever loss you experienced. (See Seek Support in chapter 6 for how to locate one)

✦ Ask a friend or partner to sit with you and let you talk about it, or bring it up in therapy.

✦ Write. Describe your grief, what you miss, what you need.

✦ Watch sad movies or read sad books.

✦ Imagine you're having a conversation with whoever you need to—e.g., the person you lost, yourself at a younger age, or yourself now. You can do this in your mind or write it as a letter that you don't mail.

✦ Ask yourself questions to evoke the feelings:

  ✦ How has this loss changed me?

  ✦ What do I miss?

  ✦ What would I want to hear?

  ✦ How can I create a new life?

  ✦ What is hardest for me in this loss?

Growth Exercise: *Accept*

An important emotional skill is how to accept—to let go—rather than keep fighting for something unattainable. In AA, the slogan "Let go and let God" is used. There's even a psychotherapy called *acceptance therapy*, devoted to this idea (Blackledge and Hayes 2001). Acceptance could also be called "letting go of an illusion," because when you accept, you're giving up a wish, hope, or dream you held dear.

An example: You've tried to please your mother your whole life, but she always criticizes you. You've tried talking to her about it, changing your communication style, being assertive. You feel you've tried everything and nothing works. You're so hurt. It's like a setup—each time you hope she'll be different, but she's not. At some point, you decide to accept rather than keep hoping for what may never be. You'll maintain a relationship with her, but you stop trying to please her. You can see that nothing you do will ever be good enough.

It will feel painful. You're accepting that you won't get the nurturing mother you always wanted. The loss of any illusion is difficult. You'll need to mourn and let yourself work through the feelings (see the growth exercise Mourn earlier in the chapter). It's never easy to let go of something you want. Indeed, some people go their whole lives hanging on to the unattainable rather than face these painful feelings.

Many wishes are attainable. But when repeated efforts prove you can't get something, it's better to accept. How can you tell when? It comes down to your degree of power over the situation. For example, there are some things over which you have control. This includes your recovery from addiction (i.e., there are always ways you can work on it). It also includes situations such as firing an employee who's doing poor work (if you're the boss) and setting limits with your children. In other situations, you don't have control. For example, you can't force your partner to stop drinking and you can't make a parent apologize for abusing you. Finally, other situations could go either way. In the example above, your efforts may have led to your mother acting differently. This is reasonable to try. But after trying everything within your power for a long time, it would appear best to finally admit she won't change. You can then move on. You are freed up to find real sources of support, rather than constantly having your hopes dashed.

How?

This growth exercise has four steps: find what you need to accept; give yourself permission to accept it; notice your feelings; and move on.

Step I: Find What You Need to Accept

Is there something you need to accept? An expectation of someone? Wanting something that is unattainable? It might feel like it's just on the edge of consciousness, as if part of you knows deep down that it's something to accept. It might be something you've been holding on to for a long time, where it feels like you keep "banging your head against a wall."

One of the most common illusions in addiction is, "I can use and it won't be a problem." You find that it always ends in disaster—one drink becomes ten—but you keep pretending it'll be different next time. Another common one for women is the illusion that an uncaring, irresponsible, or abusive partner will change: "If I just love him enough, he'll stop hitting me"; "It's true that he keeps having affairs, but he told me he'd stop"; "I know he hasn't had a job in three years, but he says he's looking." Other examples: "My father will acknowledge what he did to me"; "My boss will be the mentor I've always wanted." Remember, it needs to be something where you've tried repeatedly and to your fullest and the evidence keeps coming back the same.

What is it that you need to accept?

_____

_____

_____

Step II: Give Yourself Permission

How can you accept? You might say to yourself, "I can let go of this now. It's not healthy to persist in something that's never going to happen. I can move on. This will free me to direct my energy elsewhere. Growing means facing painful truths. If it were a perfect world, I could get this, but it's not. There are many good things in life, but this is one I won't be getting. It's okay to feel upset, to feel deprived. Over time, it'll be easier. I'm taking the step of letting go. It's like a feather into the wind—I can release it from my life."

Option: Some people like to create a ritual that symbolizes acceptance. For example, if you're letting go of drugs, you can throw out your drug material (dealer's phone number, pipe and matches).

How can you give yourself permission to let go?

_____

_____

_____

Step III: Notice Your Feelings

How upset are you? Often there's sadness, anger, loss, or deprivation. This is normal. If you want, write how it feels.

_____

_____

_____

Step IV: Move On: Replace What You've Lost

It's important to compensate for the loss. What might fill the empty space? You could choose a treat (such as a day trip, a new journal to write in, or eating out at a nice restaurant). You could find ways to bring new people into your life (e.g., join a club, take a class). Or you could write about the gifts that may come from acceptance (such as being able to spend your time and energy elsewhere). What might help you?

_____

_____

_____

Self-Awareness Summary

You can use this guide to remember the skills you want to keep learning.

How much do you *currently* use these coping skills?

	Not at all	A little	Moderately	Extremely
Soothe yourself	0	1	2	3
Choose self-respect	0	1	2	3
Mourn	0	1	2	3
Accept	0	1	2	3

How helpful would it be to use these coping skills *more*?

	Not at all helpful	A little helpful	Moderately helpful	Extremely helpful
Soothe yourself	0	1	2	3
Choose self-respect	0	1	2	3
Mourn	0	1	2	3
Accept	0	1	2	3

CHAPTER 10

Advice for the Journey

People may give up addiction out of fear, but they heal out of love.

—Charlotte Kasl, *Many Roads, One Journey*

We've reached the end, though the hope, of course, is that this is just a beginning.

The true test of an education, it's said, is being alone in a train station somewhere—you've missed your train and have several hours before the next one; there's nothing to distract you. It's just you with yourself: *What do you think about?*

My hope is that when you're sitting there, you'll have a lot of places within yourself that can give you joy, that can like yourself, that can sit with whatever comes up and find something of value in it. This is more than just not using a substance. It's about transforming yourself from someone with the self-hatred of addiction to the self-respect of someone who can face life without the false numbing of a substance. Many people have written about recovery as transformation—telling a new story, creating a new identity, attaining a higher consciousness. Most simply, it's about coming alive. If addiction means "unaware," "unconscious," "unknown," recovery means waking up.

You may wonder whether you have it in you to do this work. You may begin and soon think, "I must be doing it wrong. It's not working. I don't feel better. I've been addicted a long time, and can't change. Maybe others can, but I can't." You feel "out of shape" and want to give up. You feel overwhelmed, not knowing where to begin. Then, even though it feels this way, even though all these doubts come up, you just keep doing *something* to move forward. It feels hopeless, but you do it anyway. And you keep doing this no matter how many times you slip and fall back into using. You just keep trying. As they say, recovery is a verb.

"The doors stood open, but the captives had forgotten how to get out," Edith Wharton wrote (McKenna 1998, 74). In many ways, that is addiction. You really do have the key, you really can unlock that door, you can walk through it. You simply have to decide that you want your life back.

This holds too for the variety of problems you may be struggling with—stress, divorce, money, children, depression, anxiety, relationships, work, aging, sex, illness, discrimination, domestic violence. Whatever you face, the idea is to cope. No matter what happens, you can find a healthy way to respond.

In this book, we focused on two topics. The first was exploring your patterns—taking a deep-down look at your addiction and the life issues connected with it. The second was healing—finding ways to grow. For all the topics discussed, there could be hundreds more, equally important. Hopefully, you'll keep searching for new ways to explore, new methods of healing. It's a continual task, but likely some of the most important work you could possibly do. People who have overcome addiction say it's one of the major achievements of their lives. They are proud of it. View your recovery as a precious possession: it belongs to you. And once you've gotten yourself on solid ground, help others up that slope; as Toni Morrison said, "The function of freedom is to free someone else" (Lamott 1994, 193).

If I had to set down the key messages of this book, they would be these:

✦ There's no one right way; there's your way.

✦ Your addiction is not "who you are"; it's a problem that needs help.

✦ All feelings are important.

✦ Women are to be respected.

✦ Start early.

✦ You're a good person who's gone off track.

✦ Listen to what your behavior is telling you.

✦ Addictions are more deadly for women.

✦ Look within.

✦ Addiction is a misguided attempt to get something.

✦ The knowledge is within you.

✦ Get help for emotional problems.

✦ You have choices.

Now, how about you? As a last exercise, write down your advice to yourself. That is, after all, what counts most in the end.

_____

_____

_____

_____

_____

_____

_____

_____

_____

APPENDIX

Self-Test

Multiple Choice

If you want, take this quiz to review some of the material in this book. It's designed to be challenging, but remember, this isn't school: there's no pressure. Page numbers are provided in the Answers section to show where the information was covered. The term "addiction" refers to substance addiction.

Enjoy!

1. If you have an emotional problem and an addiction, the best advice is to work on:

    a) The addiction

    b) The emotional problem

    c) Both

    d) Whichever came first

2. Women's "telescoped course" of drinking means:

    a) Women can learn to use telescopes if they drink

    b) Drinking is a downward spiral for women

    c) Women have problems from drinking sooner than men

    d) Women have problems from drinking later than men

3. What number of drinks per day causes serious health problems for women?

    a) 1

    b) 2

    c) 3

    d) 4

4. What number of drinks per day causes serious health problems for men?

    a) 2

    b) 3

    c) 4

    d) 5

5. A key theme in this book is:

    a) What comes around goes around

    b) Choose self-respect

    c) Location, location, location

    d) Pace yourself

6. Which women have the highest rate of addiction?

    a) Whites

    b) Blacks

    c) Hispanics

    d) All three are equal

7. For women, *binge drinking* means how many drinks at a time?

   a) 2

   b) 4

   c) 6

   d) When you've lost count

8. Controlled drinking is *not* safe for:

   a) Women

   b) Air traffic controllers

   c) People with a history of alcohol dependence

   d) People with a history of drug use

9. The single best treatment for addiction is:

   a) AA

   b) Psychotherapy

   c) A combination of AA and psychotherapy

   d) There is no single best treatment

10. Which coping skill is *not* part of this book?

    a) Tell a secret

    b) Get ready

    c) Rethink

    d) Accept

11. Who has the highest rate of addiction: women or men?

    a) Women

    b) Men

    c) They are equal

    d) No one knows

12. What's the difference between mourning and depression?

    a) Mourning is healthy, depression is an illness

    b) Depression is healthy, mourning is an illness

    c) Mourning means "pain," depression means "sadness"

    d) There's no difference

13. The best definition of addiction is:

    a) How much denial you have

    b) Continued use despite harm

    c) Amount you use

    d) Level of physical dependence

14. In the U.S., what percent of people get addicted to a substance in their lifetime?
    a) 9%
    b) 15%
    c) 26%
    d) 43%

15. Who is most likely to die from addiction: women or men?
    a) Women
    b) Men
    c) They are equal
    d) Neither

16. *Harm reduction* means:
    a) Abstinence
    b) Controlled use
    c) Stress management
    d) Decreased use

17. *Trauma* is common among women; it means:
    a) Physical harm
    b) Thrill-seeking
    c) Mourning
    d) Drug dreams

18. Men are more likely than women to:
    a) Seek treatment for addiction
    b) Become addicted slowly
    c) Get support for entering addiction treatment
    d) All of the above

19. To recover from addiction, you have to:
    a) Attend AA
    b) Hit bottom
    c) Call yourself an addict
    d) None of the above

20. The most common psychiatric disorder in the U.S. is:
    a) Depression
    b) Foot fetish
    c) Substance addiction
    d) Anxiety

21. *Rethinking* means:
    a) Seeking support
    b) Positive thinking
    c) Balanced thinking
    d) Saying "Don't worry, be happy"

22. The number one cause of relapse is:
    a) Stress
    b) Thrill-seeking
    c) Body image
    d) Depression

True/False

1. As you get clean from substances, your co-occurring emotional disorder will most likely go away.   True / False

2. Most people get help for their emotional problems. True / False

3. If you have an addiction, your children are more likely to develop an addiction. True / False

4. People who attend addiction treatment voluntarily do better than those who are forced into treatment (e.g., by courts). True / False

5. Girls start drinking at a later age than boys. True / False

6. Lesbians have higher rates of addiction than straight women. True / False

7. As minorities become "acculturated" (adapt to the dominant culture) their addiction rate increases. True / False

8. Taking a psychiatric medication is the same as using a substance.
True / False

9. Successful mourning after a loss takes at least six months. True / False

10. Co-occurring disorders are more common in women than men. True / False

Answers

Multiple choice:
1. c (page 78).
2. c (pages 10–11).
3. b (page 11).
4. d (page 11).
5. b (page 162).
6. a (page 17).
7. b (page 22).
8. c (pages 42–43).
9. d (page 43).
10. b.
11. b (page 9).
12. a (page 166).
13. b (page 32).
14. c (page 16).
15. a (page 10).
16. d (page 42).
17. a (page 70).
18. d (pages 10–11, 13).
19. d (page 39, 43, 49).
20. c (page 17).
21. c (page 138).
22. a (page 60).

True / False
1. False (page 98)
2. False (page 78)
3. True (page 41)
4. False (page 49)
5. False (page 13)
6. True (page 20)
7. True (page 21)
8. False (page 49)
9. False (page 166)
10. True (page 78)

References

APA (American Psychiatric Association). 1994. *Diagnostic and Statistical Manual of Mental Disorders, 4th ed.* (DSM-IV). Washington, D.C.: American Psychiatric Association.

Battle, C., C. Zlotnick, L. M. Najavits, M. Gutierrez, and C. Winsor. In press. Posttraumatic stress disorder and substance use disorder among incarcerated women. In *Posttraumatic Stress Disorder and Substance Use Disorder*, edited by P. Ouimette and P. Brown. Washington, D.C.: American Psychological Association Press.

Beck, A. T., F. D. Wright, C. F. Newman, and B. S. Liese. 1993. *Cognitive Therapy of Substance Abuse*. New York: Guilford.

Beckman, L. J., and H. Amaro. 1986. Personal and social difficulties faced by women and men entering alcoholism treatment. *Journal of Studies on Alcohol* 47:135-145.

Blackledge, J. T., and S. C. Hayes. 2001. Emotion regulation in acceptance and commitment therapy. *Journal of Clinical Psychology* 57(2):243-255.

Blum, T., and P. Roman. 1997. Employment and drinking. In *Gender and Alcohol: Individual and Social Perspectives*, edited by R. Wilsnack and S. Wilsnack. New Brunswick, N.J.: Rutgers Center of Alcohol Studies.

Blume, S. 1998. Addictive disorders in women. In *Clinical Textbook of Addictive Disorders*, 2nd ed., edited by R. Frances and S. Miller. New York: Guilford.

———. 1997a. Women and alcohol: Issues in social policy. In *Gender and Alcohol: Individual and Social Perspectives*, edited by R. Wilsnack and S. Wilsnack. New Brunswick, N.J.: Rutgers Center of Alcohol Studies.

———. 1997b. Women: Clinical aspects. In *Substance Abuse: A Comprehensive Textbook*, 3rd ed., edited by J. Lowinson, P. Ruiz, R. Millman, and J. Langrod. Baltimore, Md.: Williams and Wilkins.

Blumenthal, S. 1998. Welcome from the U.S. Public Health Service. In *Drug Addiction Research and the Health of Women: Executive Summary*, edited by C. Wetherington and A. Roman. Rockville, Md.: U.S. Department of Health and Human Services: National Institute on Drug Abuse.

Boyd, C. J., and B. Guthrie. 1996. Women, their significant others, and crack cocaine. *American Journal on Addictions* 5(2):156-166.

Boyd, M. R., and E. J. Hauenstein. 1997. Psychiatric assessment and confirmation of dual disorders in rural substance abusing women. *Archives of Psychiatric Nursing* 11(2):74-81.

Brady, K. T., and C. L. Randall. 1999. Gender differences in substance use disorders. *Psychiatric Clinics of North America*, 22(2):241-252.

Breslau, N., R. C. Kessler, H. D. Chilcoat, L. R. Schultz, G. C. Davis, and P. Andreski. 1998. Trauma and posttraumatic stress disorder in the community: The 1996 Detroit Area Survey of Trauma. *Archives of General Psychiatry* 55(7):626-632.

Brody, J. E. 1998. A fatal shift in cancer's gender gap. *New York Times*, May 12.

Brook, J. 1998. Childhood and adolescent precursors to drug use. In *Drug Addiction Research and the Health of Women: Executive Summary*, edited by C. Wetherington and A. Roman. Rockville, Md.: U.S. Department of Health and Human Services: National Institute on Drug Abuse.

Brooner, R. K., V. L. King, M. Kidorf, C. W. Schmidt, and G. E. Bigelow. 1997. Psychiatric and substance use comorbidity among treatment-seeking opioid abusers. *Archives of General Psychiatry* 54:71-80.

Brown, P. J., R. L. Stout, and J. Gannon Rowley. 1998. Substance use disorder-PTSD comorbidity: Patients' perceptions of symptom interplay and treatment issues. *Journal of Substance Abuse Treatment* 15:5-448.

Bulik, C. M., and P. F. Sullivan. 1998. Comorbidity of eating disorders and substance-related disorders. In *Dual Diagnosis and Treatment: Substance Abuse and Comorbid Medical and Psychiatric Disorders*, edited by H. R. Kranzler and B. J. Rounsaville. New York: Marcel Dekker.

Chang, G. 1997. Primary care: Detection of women with alcohol use disorders. *Harvard Review of Psychiatry* 4(6):334-337.

Chapman, T. M. 1998. An investigation of risk factors for hidden alcohol abuse among adults with physical disabilities. Dissertation Abstracts International: Section B: The Sciences and Engineering. 59(3B):1362.

Cisler, R. A., and J. W. Nawrocki. 1998. Coping and short-term outcomes among dependent drinkers: Preliminary evidence for enhancing traditional treatment with relapse prevention training. *Alcoholism Treatment Quarterly* 16(4):5-20.

Clark, H. W. 2001. Residential substance abuse treatment for pregnant and postpartum women and their children: Treatment and policy implications. *Child Welfare* 80(2):179-198.

Coletti, S. 1998. Service provider/treatment access issues. In *Drug Addiction Research and the Health of Women: Executive Summary*, edited by C. Wetherington and A. Roman. Rockville, Md.: U.S. Department of Health and Human Services: National Institute on Drug Abuse.

Coletti, S., J. Schinka, P. Hughes, N. Hamilton, C. Renard, D. Sicilian, and R. Neri. 1997. Specialized therapeutic community treatment for chemically dependent women and their children. In *Community as Method: Therapeutic Communities for Special Populations and Special Settings*, edited by G. De Leon. Westport, Conn.: Praeger.

Combs Lane, A. M. 2001. *Risk factors associated with sexual revictimization in college women.* Dissertation Abstracts International: Section B: The Sciences and Engineering. 61(9B):4976.

Connors, G. J., S. A. Maisto, and W. H. Zywiak. 1998. Male and female alcoholics' attributions regarding the onset and termination of relapses and the maintenance of abstinence. *Journal of Substance Abuse* 101:27-42.

Cottler, L. 1998. Psychiatric sequelae of drug abuse. In *Drug Addiction Research and the Health of Women: Executive Summary*, edited by C. Wetherington and A. Roman. Rockville, Md.: U.S. Department of Health and Human Services: National Institute on Drug Abuse.

Covey, S. 1990. *The 7 Habits of Highly Effective People.* New York: Simon and Schuster.

Covington, S. S. 2000. Helping women recover: A comprehensive integrated treatment model. *Alcoholism Treatment Quarterly* 18(3):99-111.

———. 1999. *Helping Women Recover: A Program for Treating Addiction*. San Francisco: Jossey-Bass.

———. 1994. *A Woman's Way Through the Twelve Steps*. Centre City, Minn.: Hazelden.

———. 1988. *Leaving the Enchanted Forest: The Path from Relationship Addiction to Intimacy*. New York: HarperTrade.

Covington, S. S., and J. Surrey. 1997. The relational model of women's psychological development: Implications for substance abuse. In *Gender and Alcohol: Individual and Social Perspectives*, edited by R. Wilsnack and S. Wilsnack. New Brunswick, N.J.: Rutgers Center of Alcohol Studies.

CSAT (Center for Substance Abuse Treatment). in press. *Treatment Improvement Protocol: Assessment and Treatment of Persons with Co-Occurring Disorders* Rockville, Md.: U.S. Department of Health and Human Services.

———. 1994a. *Practical Approaches in the Treatment of Women Who Abuse Alcohol and Other Drugs* Rockville, Md.: Department of Health and Human Services.

———. 1994b. *Treatment Improvement Protocol: Assessment and Treatment of Patients with Coexisting Mental Illness and Alcohol and Other Drug Abuse*, vol. 9. Rockville, Md.: U.S. Department of Health and Human Services.

Curtis, G. C., W. J. Magee, W. W. Eaton, H. U. Wittchen, and R. C. Kessler. 1998. Specific fears and phobias: Epidemiology and classification. *British Journal of Psychiatry* 173:212-217.

Drug Strategies. 1998. *Keeping Score—Women and Drugs: Looking at the Federal Drug Control Budget*. Washington, D.C.: Drug Strategies.

Fillmore, K. M., J. M. Golding, E. V. Leino, M. Motoyoshi, C. Shoemaker, H. Terry, C. R. Ager, and H. P. Ferrer. 1997. Patterns and trends in women's and men's drinking. In *Gender and Alcohol: Individual and Social Perspectives*, edited by R. Wilsnack and S. Wilsnack. New Brunswick, N.J.: Rutgers Center of Alcohol Studies.

Finkelstein, N. 1993. Treatment programming for alcohol and drug-dependent pregnant women. *International Journal of the Addictions* 28(13):1275-1309.

Fletcher, A. 2001. *Sober for Good: New Solutions for Drinking Problems—Advice from Those Who Have Succeeded*. Boston: Houghton Mifflin.

Fraser, K. 1996. *Ornament and Silence: Essays on Women's Lives from Edith Wharton to Germaine Greer*. New York: Alfred Knopf.

Freud, S. 1917/1957. *Mourning and Melancholia, A General Selection from the Works of Sigmund Freud.* edited by J. Rickman. New York: Doubleday.

Gallegos, K., and G. Talbott. 1997. Physicians and other health professionals. In *Substance Abuse: A Comprehensive Textbook,* 3rd ed., edited by J. Lowinson, P. Ruiz, R. Millman, and J. Langrod. Baltimore, Md.: Williams and Wilkins.

Glick, J., and D. Halperin. 1997. Collection and accumulation. In *Substance Abuse: A Comprehensive Textbook,* 3rd ed., edited by J. Lowinson, P. Ruiz, R. Millman, and J. Langrod. Baltimore, Md.: Williams and Wilkins.

Gold, M., C. Johnson, and K. Stennie. 1997. Eating disorders. In *Substance Abuse: A Comprehensive Textbook,* Third Edition, edited by J. Lowinson, P. Ruiz, R. Millman, and J. Langrod. Baltimore, Md.: Williams and Wilkins.

Goldberg, N. 2002. *Women Are Not Small Men: Life-Saving Strategies for Preventing and Healing Heart Disease in Women.* New York: Ballantine.

Gomberg, E. 1997. Alcohol abuse: Age and gender differences. In *Gender and Alcohol: Individual and Social Perspectives,* edited by R. Wilsnack and S. Wilsnack. New Brunswick, N.J.: Rutgers Center of Alcohol Studies.

Gomberg, E., and T. Nirenberg. 1993. Antecedents and consequences. In *Women and Substance Abuse,* edited by E. Gomberg and T. Nirenberg. Norwood, N.J.: Ablex.

Goode, M. 1999. *The Land Before Time.* New York: Random House.

Goodman, A. 1997. Sexual addiction. In *Substance Abuse: A Comprehensive Textbook,* 3rd ed., edited by J. Lowinson, P. Ruiz, R. Millman, and J. Langrod. Baltimore, Md.: Williams and Wilkins.

Graham, K., and K. Braun. 1999. Concordance of use of alcohol and other substances among older adult couples. *Addictive Behaviors* 24(6):839-856.

Grant, B. F. 1997. Prevalence and correlates of alcohol use and DSM-IV alcohol dependence in the United States: Results of the National Longitudinal Alcohol Epidemiologic Survey. *Journal of Studies on Alcohol* 58(5):464-473.

Greenfield, S. 2002. Personal communication, February 1.

———. 2002. Women and alcohol use disorders. *Harvard Review of Psychiatry* 10:76–85.

Greenfield, S. and G. O'Leary. In press- a. Gender Differences in Substance Use Disorders. In *Psychiatric Illness in Women: Emerging Treatments and Research,* edited by F. Lewis-Hall, J. Herrera, and Eli Lilly and Company. Washington, D.C.: American Psychiatric Press, Inc.

Heath, D. 1993. Cross-cultural perspectives on women and alcohol. In *Women and Substance Abuse,* edited by E. Gomberg and T. Nirenberg. Norwood, N.J.: Ablex.

Heinemann, A. 1997. Persons with disabilities. In *Substance Abuse: A Comprehensive Textbook,* 3rd ed., edited by J. Lowinson, P. Ruiz, R. Millman, and J. Langrod. Baltimore, Md.: Williams and Wilkins.

Henderson, D. J. 1998. Drug abuse and incarcerated women: A research review. *Journal of Substance Abuse Treatment* 15(6):579-587.

Hien, D., and N. M. Hien. 1998. Women, violence with intimates and substance abuse: Relevant theory, empirical findings, and recommendations for future research. *American Journal of Drug and Alcohol Abuse* 24(3):419-438.

Hughes, L. 1994. From *The Collected Poems of Langston Hughes,* edited by A. Rampersad and D. Roessel. New York: Alfred A. Knopf.

James, W. 1902/1958. *The Varieties of Religious Experience: A Study in Human Nature.* New York: Mentor.

Jordan, J., I. Stiver, A. Kaplan, J. Miller, and J. Surrey. 1991. *Women's Growth in Connection: Writings from the Stone Center.* New York: Guilford.

Jumper-Thurman, P. 1998. Research needs of American Indian women. In *Drug Addiction Research and the Health of Women: Executive Summary,* edited by C. Wetherington and A. Roman. Rockville, Md.: U.S. Department of Health and Human Services: National Institute on Drug Abuse.

Kandall, S. 1998. The history of drug abuse and women in the United States. In *Drug Addiction Research and the Health of Women: Executive Summary*, edited by C. Wetherington and A. Roman. Rockville, Md.: U.S. Department of Health and Human Services: National Institute on Drug Abuse.

Kandel, D. 1998. Epidemiology of drug use and abuse among women. In *Drug Addiction Research and the Health of Women: Executive Summary*, edited by C. Wetherington and A. Roman. Rockville, Md.: U.S. Department of Health and Human Services: National Institute on Drug Abuse.

Karpman, B. 1956. *The Alcoholic Woman.* Washington, D.C.: Linacre Press.

Kaskutas, L. A. 1996. Predictors of self esteem among members of Women For Sobriety. *Addiction Research* 4:273–281.

Kasl, C. 1992. *Many Roads, One Journey.* New York: HarperPerennial.

Kasl, C. 1990. *Women, Sex, and Addictions: A Search for Love and Power.* New York: HarperTrade.

Kendler, K. S., C. G. Davis, and R. C. Kessler. 1997. The familial aggregation of common psychiatric and substance use disorders in the National Comorbidity Survey: A family history study. *British Journal of Psychiatry* 170:541-548.

Kessler, R. C., R. C. Crum, L. A. Warner, C. B. Nelson, J. Schulenberg, and J. C. Anthony. 1997. Lifetime co-occurence of DSM-III-R alcohol abuse and dependence with other psychiatric disorders in the National Comorbidity Survey. *Archives of General Psychiatry* 54:313-321.

Kessler, R. C., K. A. McGonagle, S. Zhao, C. B. Nelson, M. Hughes, S. Eshleman, H.-U. Wittchen, and K. S. Kendler. 1994. Lifetime and 12-month prevalence of DSM-III-R psychiatric disorders in the United States: Results from the national comorbidity survey. *Archives of General Psychiatry* 51:8-19.

Kessler, R. C., C. B. Nelson, K. A. McGonagle, M. J. Edlund, R. G. Frank, and P. J. Leaf. 1996. The epidemiology of co-occurring addictive and mental disorders: Implications for prevention and service utilization. *American Journal of Orthopsychiatry* 66(1):17-31.

Kessler, R. C., A. Sonnega, E. Bromet, M. Hughes, and C. B. Nelson. 1995. Posttraumatic stress disorder in the national comorbidity survey. *Archives of General Psychiatry* 52:1048-1060.

Khantzian, E. J. 1997. The self-medication hypothesis of substance use disorders: A reconsideration and recent applications. *Harvard Review of Psychiatry* 4:231-244.

Kilbourne, J. 2002. *Deadly persuasion: Advertising and Addiction.* Paper presented at the Cambridge Hospital conference, "25 Years of Addiction Treatment," Boston. February.

Killeen, T., and K. T. Brady. 2000. Parental stress and child behavioral outcomes following substance abuse residential treatment: Follow-up at 6 and 12 months. *Journal of Substance Abuse Treatment* 19(1)23-29.

Kilpatrick, D., H. Resnick, B. Saunders, and C. Best. 1998. Victimization, posttraumatic stress disorder, and substance use/abuse among women. In *Drug Addiction Research and the Health of Women (NIH Publication No. 98-4290)*, edited by C. L. Wetherington and A. B. Roman. Rockville, Md.: U.S. Department of Health and Human Services. National Institute on Drug Abuse.

Knapp, C. 1997. *Drinking: A Love Story*. New York: Bantam.

Knowlton, L. 1995. Public and research views of dual-diagnosis. *Psychiatric Times*, 12(5) May.

Kouzekanani, K., and M. A. Neeley. 1997. Coping styles of female cocaine addicts. *Substance Abuse* 18(4):165-171.

Lamott, A. 1994. *Bird by Bird: Some Instructions on Writing and Life*. New York: Random House.

Leshner, A. 1999. *Substance Abuse.* Paper presented at the National Center for Responsible Gaming Conference "New Directions in Gambling Addiction Research," Washington, D.C.

Lewin, K. 1951. *Field Theory in Social Science*. New York: Harper & Brothers.

Lichtenstein, B. 1997. Women and crack-cocaine use: A study of social networks and HIV risk in an Alabama jail sample. *Addiction Research* 5(4):279-296.

Manter du Wors, G. 1992. *White Knuckles and Wishful Thinking*. Seattle: Hogrefe and Huber.

Margolis, R., and J. Zweben. 1998. *Treating Patients with Alcohol and Other Drug Problems: An Integrated Approach*. Washington, D.C.: American Psychological Association.

McCaul, M. E., and D. S. Svikis. 1999. Intervention issues for women. In *Sourcebook on Substance Abuse: Etiology, Epidemiology, Assessment, and Treatment*, edited by P. J. Ott and R. E. Tarter. Needham Heights, Mass.: Allyn and Bacon.

McCrady, B. S., and H. Raytek. 1993. Women and substance abuse: Treatment modalities and outcomes. In *Women and Substance Abuse*, edited by E. Gomberg and T. Nirenberg. Norwood, N.J.: Ablex.

McCrady, B. S., and J. W. Langenbucher. 1996. Alcohol treatment and health care system reform. *Archives of General Psychiatry* 53(8):737-746.

McKenna, E. P. 1998. *When Work Doesn't Work Anymore: Women, Work, and Identity*. New York: Bantam Doubleday Dell.

McLellan, A. T., H. Kushner, D. Metzger, R. Peters, I. Smith, G. Grissom, H. Pettinati, and M. Argeriou. 1992. The fifth edition of the Addiction Severity Index. *Journal of Substance Abuse Treatment* 9:199-213.

McLellan, A. T., G. E. Woody, L. Luborsky, and L. Goehl. 1988. Is the counselor an "active ingredient" in substance abuse rehabilitation? An examination of treatment success among four counselors. *Journal of Nervous and Mental Disease* 176:423-430.

Mendelson, J. H., and N. K. Mello. 1998. Diagnostic evaluation of alcohol and drug abuse problems in women. *Psychopharmacology Bulletin* 34(3):279-281.

Merikangas, K. 1998. The etiology and genetic epidemiology of psychiatric and drug disorders among women. In *Drug Addiction Research and the Health of Women: Executive Summary*, edited by C. Wetherington and A. Roman. Rockville, Md.: U.S. Department of Health and Human Services: National Institute on Drug Abuse.

Michels, P. J., N. P. Johnson, R. Mallin, J. T. Thornhill, S. Sharma, H. Gonzales, and R. Kellett. 1999. Coping strategies of alcoholic women. *Substance Abuse* 20(4):237-248.

Miles, D. R., M. B. M. van den Bree., A. E. Gupman, D. B. Newlin, M. D. Glantz, and R. W. Pickens. 2001. A twin study on sensation seeking, risk taking behavior and marijuana use. *Drug and Alcohol Dependence* 62(1):57-68.

Miller, A. L. 1999. *Stress, Coping and Social Support: Strategies Among Female Substance Abusers.* Dissertation Abstracts International Section A: Humanities and Social Sciences. 59(7A):2721.

Miller, B., W. Downs, and M. Testa. 1993. Interrelationships between victimization experiences and women's alcohol use. *Journal of Studies on Alcohol* 54(Suppl 11):109-117.

Miller, L., A. D. Smith, and L. Rothstein. 1993. *The Stress Solution: An Action Plan to Manage Stress in Your Life.* New York: Simon and Schuster.

Miller, W., J. Brown, T. Simpson, N. Handmaker, T. Bein, L. Luckie, H. Montgomery, R. Hester, and J. Tonigan. 1995. What works? A methodological analysis of the alcohol treatment outcome literature. In *Handbook of Alcoholism Treatment Approaches: Effective Alternatives*, edited by R. Hester and W. Miller. Boston: Allyn and Bacon.

Miller, W. R., and A. C. Page. 1991. Warm turkey: Other routes to abstinence. *Journal of Substance Abuse Treatment* 8:227-232.

Moras, K. 1998. Psychosocial and behavioral treatments for women. In *Drug Addiction Research and the Health of Women: Executive Summary*, edited by C. Wetherington and A. Roman. Rockville, Md.: U.S. Department of Health and Human Services: National Institute on Drug Abuse.

Mullings, J. L. 1998. *Victimization, Substance Abuse, and High Risk Behavior as Predictors of Health Among Women at Admission to Prison.* Dissertation Abstracts International Section A: Humanities and Social Sciences. 58(9A):3730.

Nadeau, L., and K. Harvey. 1995. Women's alcoholic intoxication: The origins of the double standard in Canada. *Addiction Research* 2(3):279-290.

Najavits, L. M. 2002. *Seeking Safety: A Treatment Manual for PTSD and Substance Abuse.* New York: Guilford.

Najavits, L. M., P. Crits-Christoph, and A. Dierberger. 2000. Clinicians' impact on the quality of substance use disorder treatment. *Substance Use and Misuse* 35(12-14):2161-2190.

Najavits, L. M., and R. D. Weiss. 1994. The role of psychotherapy in the treatment of substance use disorders. *Harvard Review of Psychiatry* 2:84-96.

Najavits, L. M., R. D. Weiss, and S. R. Shaw. 1997. The link between substance abuse and posttraumatic stress disorder in women: A research review. *American Journal on Addictions* 6(4):273-283.

Najavits, L. M., F. Abueg, P. Brown, B. Dansky, T. Keane, and J. Lovern. 1998. *Numbing the Pain*. Nevada City, Calif.: Cavalcade Productions.

NCHS (National Center for Health Statistics). 2001. Health, United States, 2001, With Urban and Rural Health Chartbook. U.S. Department of Health and Human Services: Centers for Disease Control. www.cdc.gov/nchs/products/pubs/pubd/hus/hus.htm.

NFDI (National Foundation for Depressive Illness). 2001. Now we can successfully treat the illness called depression. Downloaded 1/10/02 from www.depression.org

NIAAA (National Institute on Alcohol Abuse and Alcoholism). 2001. Frequently asked questions. Downloaded 11/01 from www.niaaa.nih.gov/faq/q-a.htm.

NIDA (National Institute on Drug Abuse). 2001. *Stress and substance abuse: A special report*. Downloaded 11/5/01 from www.nida.nih.gov/stressanddrugabuse.html

———. 2000. Gender differences in drug abuse risks and treatment. *NIDA Notes* 15:15.

———. 1999. Principles of Drug Addiction Treatment: A Research-Based Guide. National Institute of Health Publication No. 99–4180. Bethesda, Md.: National Institute on Drug Abuse.

NIMH (National Institute of Mental Health). 2000. Depression. National Institutes of Health Publication No. 00-3561. Bethesda, Md.: National Institute of Mental Health.

Nelson, C. B., A. C. Heath, and R. C. Kessler. 1998. Temporal progression of alcohol dependence symptoms: Results from the national comorbidity survey. *Journal of Consulting and Clinical Psychology* 66(3):474-483.

Paltrow, L. 1998. Punishing women for their behavior during pregnancy: An approach that undermines the health of women and children. In *Drug Addiction Research and the Health of Women: Executive Summary*, edited by C. Wetherington and A. Roman. Rockville, Md.: U.S. Department of Health and Human Services: National Institute on Drug Abuse.

Peters, R. H., A. L. Strozier, M. R. Murrin, and W. D. Kearns. 1997. Treatment of substance-abusing jail inmates: Examination of gender differences. *Journal of Substance Abuse Treatment* 14(4):339-349.

Piazza, N., J. Vrbka, and R. Yeager. 1989. Telescoping of alcoholism in women alcoholics. *International Journal of Addiction* 24:19-28.

Pierce, E. F., K. A. Rohaly, and B. Fritchley. 1997. Sex differences on exercise dependence for men and women in a marathon road race. *Perceptual and Motor Skills* 84: 991-994.

Plumb, M. 1998. Drug abuse and HIV among lesbians. In *Drug Addiction Research and the Health of Women: Executive Summary*, edited by C. Wetherington and A. Roman. Rockville, Md.: U.S. Department of Health and Human Services: National Institute on Drug Abuse.

Powell, J., K. Hardoon, J. L. Derevensky, and R. Gupta. 1999. Gambling and risk-taking behavior among university students. *Substance Use and Misuse* 34(8):1167-1184.

Putnam, R. D. 2000. *Bowling Alone: The Collapse and Revival of American Community.* New York: Simon and Schuster.

Regier, D. A., M. E. Farmer, D. S. Rae, B. Z. Locke, S. J. Keith, L. L. Judd, and F. K. Goodwin. 1990. Co-morbidity of mental disorders with alcohol and other drug abuse: Results from the Epidemiologic Catchment Area (ECA) study. *Journal of the American Medical Association* 264:2511-2518.

Rhodes, R., and A. Johnson. 1997. A feminist approach to treating alcohol and drug-addicted African-American women. *Women and Therapy* 20(3):23-37.

Rich, M. 1998. *Women Who Gamble.* Dissertation Abstracts International: Section B: The Sciences and Engineering. 581(2B):6823.

Rosenheck, R. A. 1999. Principles for priority setting in mental health services and their implications for the least well off. *Psychiatric Services* 50(5):653-658.

Rubin, A., R. L. Stout, and R. Longabaugh. 1996. Section IIA. Replication and extension of Marlatt's taxonomy: Gender differences in relapse situations. *Addiction* (91)Suppl:S11–S120

Ruzek, J. I., M. A. Polusny, and F. R. Abueg. 1998. Assessment and treatment of concurrent posttraumatic stress disorder and substance abuse. In *Cognitive-Behavioral Therapies for Trauma*, edited by V. M. Follett, J. I. Ruzek, and F. R. Abueg. New York: Guilford.

SAMHSA (Substance Abuse and Mental Health Services Administration). 2001a. *A Provider's Introduction to Substance Abuse Treatment for Lesbian, Gay, Bisexual, and Transgender Individuals.* Rockville, Md.: U.S. Department of Health and Human Services: Substance Abuse and Mental Health Services Administration.

———. 2001b. *Summary of Findings from the 2000 National Household Survey on Drug Abuse.* Rockville, Md.: U.S. Department of Health and Human Services: Substance Abuse and Mental Health Services Administration.

———. 1998. *Services Research Outcomes Study.* Rockville, Md.: Substance Abuse and Mental Health Services Administration.

———. 1997. *National Treatment Improvement Evaluation Study.* Rockville, Md.: Substance Abuse and Mental Health Services Administration.

Sanders-Phillips, K. 1998. Intervention, outreach, and special needs. In *Drug Addiction Research and the Health of Women: Executive Summary*, edited by C. Wetherington and A. Roman. Rockville, Md.: U.S. Department of Health and Human Services: National Institute on Drug Abuse.

Schellenberg, J. A. 1998. *Transpersonal experiences and Practices of Women Who Are Healing Childhood Sexual Abuse.* Dissertation Abstracts International: Section B: The Sciences and Engineering. 59(5B):2433.

Schmidt, L. G., P. Dufeu, S. Kuhn, M. Smolka, and H. Rommelspacher. 2000. Transition to alcohol dependence: Clinical and neurobiological considerations. *Comprehensive Psychiatry* 41(2, Suppl 1):90-94.

Schnoll, S. 1998. Pharmacology: Sex-specific considerations in the use of psychoactive medications. In *Drug Addiction Research and the Health of Women: Executive Summary*, edited by C. Wetherington and A. Roman. Rockville, Md.: U.S. Department of Health and Human Services: National Institute on Drug Abuse.

Schober, R., and H. M. Annis. 1996. Barriers to help-seeking for change in drinking: A gender-focused review of the literature. *Addictive Behaviors* 21(1):81-92.

Schuckit, M. A. 1998. "Sex-related differences in depressed alcoholics": Dr. Schuckit replies. *American Journal of Psychiatry* 155(10):1465.

Selwyn, P. 1998. Medical and health consequences of HIV/AIDS and drug abuse. In *Drug Addiction Research and the Health of Women: Executive Summary*, edited by C. Wetherington and A. Roman. Rockville, Md.: U.S. Department of Health and Human Services: National Institute on Drug Abuse.

Shaffer, H. J. 1997. The most important unresolved issue in the addictions: Conceptual chaos. *Substance Use and Misuse* 32(11):1573-1580.

Simpson, D. D., G. W. Joe, G. A. Rowan Szal, and J. M. Greener. 1997. Drug abuse treatment process components that improve retention. *Journal of Substance Abuse Treatment* 14(6):565-572.

Tarter, R. E., L. Kirisci, and A. Mezzich. 1997. Multivariate typology of adolescents with alcohol use disorder. *American Journal on Addictions* 6(2):150-158.

Taylor, A. 1998. Needlework: The lifestyle of female drug injectors. *Journal of Drug Issues* 28(1):77-90.

Volpicelli, J., H. Pettinati, A. McLellan, and C. O'Brien. 2001. *Combining Medication and Psychosocial Treatments for Addictions: The BRENDA Approach*. New York: Guilford.

Walitzer, K., and G. Connors. 1997. Gender and treatment of alcohol-related problems. In *Gender and Alcohol: Individual and Social Perspectives*, edited by R. Wilsnack and S. Wilsnack. New Brunswick, N.J.: Rutgers Center of Alcohol Studies.

Wallen, J. 1998. Researcher/sex issues. In *Drug Addiction Research and the Health of Women: Executive Summary*, edited by C. Wetherington and A. Roman. Rockville, MD: U.S. Department of Health and Human Services: National Institute on Drug Abuse.

Weiss, R. D., J. Martinez Raga, M. L. Griffin, S. F. Greenfield, and C. Hufford. 1997. Gender differences in cocaine dependent patients: A 6-month follow-up study. *Drug and Alcohol Dependence* 44(1):35-40.

Weiss, R. D., L. M. Najavits, and S. Greenfield. 1999. A relapse prevention group for patients with bipolar and substance use disorders. *Journal of Substance Abuse Treatment* 16:47-54.

Weiss, R. D., L. M. Najavits, and S. M. Mirin. 1998. Substance abuse and psychiatric disorders. In *Clinical Textbook of Addictive Disorders*, 2nd ed., edited by R. J. Frances and S. I. Miller. New York: Guilford.

White, K. A., K. T. Brady, and S. Sonne. 1996. Gender differences in patterns of cocaine use. *American Journal on Addictions* 5(3):259-261.

Wilsnack, R., and S. Wilsnack, editors. 1997. *Gender and Alcohol: Individual and Social Perspectives*. New Brunswick, N.J.: Rutgers Center of Alcohol Studies.

Woods, J. 1998. Translating basic research into the clinical setting. In *Drug Addiction Research and the Health of Women: Executive Summary*, edited by C. Wetherington and A. Roman. Rockville, Md.: U.S. Department of Health and Human Services: National Institute on Drug Abuse.

Zweben, J. E., H. W. Clark, and D. E. Smith. 1994. Traumatic experiences and substance abuse: Mapping the territory. *Journal of Psychoactive Drugs* 26:327-344.

Lisa M. Najavits, Ph.D., is Associate Professor in the Department of Psychiatry at Harvard Medical School, Director of the Trauma Research Program in the Alcohol and Drug Abuse Treatment Center of McLean Hospital in Belmont, Massachusetts, and Chair of the Women's Initiative of Harvard Medical School's Division on Addictions. Dr. Najavits has received, as principal investigator, four National Institutes of Health research grants, including an Independent Scientist Career Award from the National Institute on Drug Abuse and three grants for treatment outcome studies on posttraumatic stress disorder and substance abuse. Author of the book Seeking Safety: A Treatment Manual for PTSD and Substance Abuse (2002) and more than 60 professional publications, she is on the advisory boards of Psychotherapy Research, the Journal of Traumatic Stress, and Clinical Psychology: Science and Practice. Dr. Najavits is past-president of the New England Society for Behavior Analysis and Therapy and was recipient of the Chaim Danieli Young Professional Award of the International Society for Traumatic Stress Studies in 1997, and the Early Career Award of the Society for Psychotherapy Research in 1998. She is a licensed psychologist who conducts a psychotherapy practice in Massachusetts. Her major clinical and research interests include substance abuse, posttraumatic stress disorder, women's mental health treatment, and psychotherapy outcome research.

Some Other
New Harbinger Titles

Watercooler Wisdom, Item 4364 $14.95

The Juicy Tomato Guide to Ripe Living After 50, Item 4321 $16.95

What's Right With Me, Item 4429 $16.95

The Balanced Mom, Item 4534 $14.95

Women Who Worry Too Much, Item 4127 $13.95

In Harm's Way, Item 4003 $14.95

Breastfeeding Made Simple, Item 4046 $16.95

The Well-Ordered Office, Item 3856 $13.95

Talk to Me, Item 3317 $12.95

Romantic Intelligence, Item 3309 $15.95

Transformational Divorce, Item 3414 $13.95

The Rape Recovery Handbook, Item 3376 $15.95

Eating Mindfully, Item 3503 $13.95

Sex Talk, Item 2868 $12.95

Everyday Adventures for the Soul, Item 2981 $11.95

A Woman's Addiction Workbook, Item 2973 $19.95

The Daughter-In-Law's Survival Guide, Item 2817 $12.95

PMDD, Item 2833 $13.95

The Vulvodynia Survival Guide, Item 2914 $16.95

Love Tune-Ups, Item 2744 $10.95

Brave New You, Item 2590 $13.95

The Woman's Book of Sleep, Item 2493 $14.95

Pregnancy Stories, Item 2361 $14.95

The Women's Guide to Total Self-Esteem, Item 2418 $14.95

The Conscious Bride, Item 2132 $12.95

Juicy Tomatoes, Item 2175 $14.95

High on Stress, Item 1101 $13.95

Perimenopause, 2nd edition, Item 2345 $17.95

The Infertility Survival Guide, Item 2477 $16.95

Call **toll free, 1-800-748-6273,** or log on to our online bookstore at **www.newharbinger.com** to order. Have your Visa or Mastercard number ready. Or send a check for the titles you want to New Harbinger Publications, Inc., 5674 Shattuck Ave., Oakland, CA 94609. Include $4.50 for the first book and 75¢ for each additional book, to cover shipping and handling. (California residents please include appropriate sales tax.) Allow two to five weeks for delivery.

Prices subject to change without notice.